women *in* overdrive

*find balance & overcome
burnout at any age*

nora isaacs

SEAL PRESS

Published by Seal Press
An Imprint of Avalon Publishing Group, Incorporated
1400 65th Street, Suite 250
AVALON
publishing group incorporated Emeryville, CA 94608

9 8 7 6 5 4 3 2 1

Library of Congress Cataloging-in-Publication Data
Isaacs, Nora.
Women in overdrive : find balance and overcome burnout at any age /
Nora Isaacs.
        p. cm.
ISBN-13: 978-1-58005-161-3
ISBN-10: 1-58005-161-8
1. Women-Mental health. 2. Burn out (Psychology)-Treatment. I. Title.

RC451.4.W6I83 2006
616.9'80082-dc22
2006021118

Book design by Kate Basart/Union Pageworks
Printed in the United States of America by Worzalla
Distributed by Publishers Group West

contents

For my grandmother, Frances, and

my mother, Faith, who live with

strength, humility, and grace.

The trouble with the rat race is that even if
you win, you're still a rat.

—Lily Tomlin

foreword

I was excited by the request to write this foreword, not only because I am friends with Nora but also because I was fascinated by the topic. The only thing that was holding me back was I just couldn't seem to find any time to do it. Either I was preparing to travel to teach a workshop, dealing with reentry after the workshop, putting energy into running my home, practicing yoga, or studying my new hobby of learning Spanish, not to mention connecting with my husband and children.

After a few weeks of procrastination it suddenly dawned on me in what I call "a blinding flash of the obvious": The reason I had no time to write the foreword for *Women in Overdrive* was that *I was in overdrive*. On further reflection, it became clear that it wasn't just me; I realized that most of my friends were there, too.

Perhaps part of the reason that so many women find ourselves in this state may very well be based paradoxically on the number of choices we have in our lives. Fifty years ago, the choices for most women were fairly limited. Most of us became wives and mothers and homemakers; even if we were college educated in rigorous academic fields, we did not work outside the home. There was a consistent routine to life. Stores were closed on Sundays and banks by 2 PM most days. The amount

of time for "work" was so much less than now—when we can
order clothes online at 11 PM and shop for food at stores open
twenty-four hours a day. These days there are almost no limits
to the time available for "doing work."

But more important, there is now a societal expectation that
women will have a demanding career beyond the phenomenal
demands inherent in being a wife and mother. While I celebrate
that we have these choices, they are just being added to other
"jobs." The expectations of experiencing motherhood and of
excelling at being a homemaker, while sometimes lessened, are
still strong and continue to be embraced by women ourselves.
We keep taking on more and more. So not only are we trying
to live up to our mothers' and grandmothers' images as full-
time homemakers, we are going to medical school and staying
physically fit at the gym and being mothers and wives as well,
not to mention working at our children's school and at our
church or volunteering in our community, all at once.

Because our choices are so many and so interesting, we seem
to feel "compelled" to make those choices. We begin to believe
that we can "have it all"—now, there is a lie if there ever was
one. While we hear and read that we can "have it all," what that
actually means is that we must let go of meeting our own needs
for the basics like space, rest, and simple uncommitted slots of
time to think and laze about. To meet all the demands of our
various roles we push ourselves, stay up too late, eat too much
or not at all, and work all the time, thinking of any car trip as
a perfect chance to do more by making calls on the cell phone.
I really know I am doing too much when I drive along and call
back to my house to leave myself messages on my home phone

to remind myself not to forget yet another errand. I have become my own assistant, thus bringing "efficiency" to a new level.

In *Women in Overdrive,* Nora Isaacs takes us through the process of what it means to be in overdrive and helps us become reacquainted with the costs we pay to stay there. She reminds us that not only do we shortchange our families, we shortchange ourselves by our constant fatigue. We are no doubt shortening our lives and damaging our health in our race to do more, produce more, and achieve more.

Carefully, Nora not only explains the costs of our choices but offers us the simple cure: We must listen more intuitively and with more trust to our inner voice and our inner needs. This book is full of compelling examples of real women who have learned by sometimes life-threatening experiences the power of doing just that. To find the balance we all crave, Nora suggests that we seek first to be rested and nutritionally and emotionally fed, and that we find a centering practice like meditation, yoga, or tai chi to stabilize our health and our emotions. These things, she states emphatically, are no longer "extras" but imperatives. She also offers suggestions for food and supplements that can soothe and ease our weariness.

But what I like most about *Women in Overdrive* is the powerful message it offers in different ways in each chapter. Women are doing too much, and that is not only taking its toll on us but is hurting our families and sadly modeling that behavior to the next generation of young women. She reminds us that we are creating a personal and social world that is full of accomplishment and material things but lacks deep satisfaction and personal peace. We are at the mercy of the belief that whatever we are doing, *it is never enough*. I especially like this quote from Chapter 9: We continually are "juggling work and home life . . . friends and responsibilities . . . our personal needs with the needs of our families. It's helpful to take a step back and to look at the benefits [of rest]: a cool head, a calm mind, and an open heart." This is how I want to live, and I am guessing you do, too.

Taking in Nora's advice about how to live and let go, I glean from her writing that while it is difficult to do less if we are addicted to accomplishment, it is definitely possible. It is the little choices that make the difference. Can we say no to the next appeal for our help, the next project, or the next committee that "desperately" needs our help? *Women in Overdrive* not only offers helpful hints about how to restore our natural rhythms, it inspires us with the reasons to do so. I hope you will enjoy the book as I did and, even more, that you will take one afternoon or even a whole day, in the midst of a world that tells us to keep moving and do more, to "just be" and to enjoy the sweetness of stillness and rest.

—Judith Hanson Lasater, PhD, PT
San Francisco, California
September 2006

introduction

Like many women I know, I've lived much of my life in over-drive. Given a choice between doing and not doing, I always chose doing. I wanted to be the best at everything. The more tasks I accomplished, the higher my self-worth. I liked to keep moving. Multitasking was my rule rather than my exception. I found comfort in perfectionism.

It was challenging for me to take time out of my day for meditation. I went out of my way to take care of people, and it was hard for me to say no. I took on more projects than I could comfortably handle and tried to be everything to everybody. At times I felt as if I were about to crack, and I knew that this status was unsustainable, especially if I wanted to remain healthy and age well.

To counter my overdrive tendencies, over the past few years I've done my best to shift gears. I've educated myself about how stress hormones work, about the connection between imbalance in the mind and disease in the body, and about ways that complementary medicine like acupuncture and massage can help. I've tried yoga, meditation, and simple breathing for anxiety. I've chosen to simplify my life rather than relentlessly pursue material possessions. I nurture friendships, relation-ships, and work that I love in order to keep myself centered.

As I've consciously tried to slow down, I've realized that overdrive is a common physical and emotional state for busy women—whether we're managing a career, family, elderly parents, or all of these things combined. We live in a culture where we aren't encouraged, either subtly or overtly, to relax or take time for ourselves. As we earn more money, take on more responsibilities, and gain more status at work, we still feel pressured to find the time to nurture our relationships, run our households, and take care of our children. It's no wonder that staying calm and relatively stress-free often falls by the wayside. Yet whether we're in our thirties or seventies, it's never too late to step out of overdrive and learn how to live more balanced, richer, and deeply connected lives.

In my conversations with women of all ages, I've found that most everyone wants more simplicity in her life—but many can't imagine a single thing that they would give up to allow for the relaxation and balance they crave. So, women in overdrive face a perplexing dilemma: We want to do everything life has to offer, but we know we need to slow down. This is the paradox I address in this book, which is the result of what I've learned through years of research, hard-won experience, and conversations with dozens of women about how they've survived and thrived. *Women in Overdrive* offers ways for women of every decade to cultivate awareness and implement strategies for not getting burned out.

We can't talk about overdrive without talking about aging. I believe that stepping out of overdrive is the key to aging well, and my own experience as the daughter of yoga teachers has given me evidence to back up this theory. A few weeks ago, my mother received a call from a national magazine. The editor—a former colleague of mine—knew my mother was a lifelong yoga practitioner, and he needed someone to model poses for an upcoming article on yoga and aging. They set up a time for a photo test, and before they hung up, he asked her to email a few photographs to show his fellow editors for a preview. The next day, he called back. With an apologetic tone, he told her she didn't need to come in after all. "It's just that . . . you just look too young," he explained. "We want someone who *looks* sixty-four."

Turns out, they wanted someone with silver hair and more slack features—the stereotypical image of a women in her sixties. But that's not my mother, who has been practicing yoga, exercising, and eating a balanced diet for decades. And she's not the only one aging well and expecting more out of life. A 2003 Rehabilitation Institute of Chicago study showed that Baby Boomers expect not only to live longer than the average life expectancy—but to remain active until the end. Fifty percent of the study's respondents said they plan on making it beyond age eighty without serious limitation on their activities, and 79 percent feel they will not experience serious limitation until beyond age seventy.[1]

These remarkable statistics show a dramatic change from previous generations. Beyond aging more gracefully, it seems that many women have made a conscious commitment *not* to age as their parents did. In my family's lineage of women, this contrast is particularly stark. My grandmother Frances—my mother's mother—seemed to me like an "old person" at sixty-four. Although she was probably only sixty when she moved into our little back room in suburban New Jersey, I thought she was ancient. She walked slowly and deliberately, suffered bouts of shortness of breath, carefully styled her white hair, and stocked the medicine cabinet full of prescription drugs. I can't remember her ever exercising—or even talking about it.

My mother, on the other hand, discovered yoga in her late twenties after having my older sister, Elana. She had always worked outside the home, and so staying in all day with an infant made her "stir crazy." She found a local yoga class and became hooked on yoga's physical benefits and its subtle yet profound effect on the mind. (My dad joined her shortly thereafter, but for less noble reasons: The young, male teacher tended to adjust his students too much for my dad's liking—especially when it was his wife on the receiving end!)

But what started as a mere diversion ended up as a lifelong journey in the exploration of alternative methods of health, including macrobiotic cooking, tai chi, ayurvedic massage, craniosacral therapy, Feldenkrais, qigong, Rolfing, vegetarianism, Chinese medicine, homeopathy, and acupuncture, as well as the exploration of many schools of faith, such as Buddhism, Jewish mysticism, Christian Science, and Hinduism. Today my mother doesn't dye her hair (it's still naturally brown), take any medication, or have any chronic health problems. She eats healthy food, regularly visits the chiropractor and masseuse, practices tai chi, and teaches yoga. Her endless stamina and physical strength rival that of any forty-year-old. Whenever she tries to get into the movies or on public transportation as a "senior," she is always met with a look of disbelief from the ticket-taker.

This discrepancy between my grandmother's and mother's aging process has opened my eyes to taking a more holistic approach to aging. As a health journalist, I've written many articles over the past five years that point to the interest in alternative ways of healing. Some of my recent assignments have covered pharmacies that integrate Eastern and Western medi-

cine; a new, nationwide chain of healing centers; and the growing trend of healthy vacations. With a passion to take charge of
our health, we are embracing complementary and alternative
medicine en masse. In addition to the physical, people are looking at the spiritual elements of staying healthy and living longer.
I often wonder if my Grandma Frances's quality of life would
have been better if she were still here today. Would she have
done yoga? Gone to an acupuncturist? Learned to meditate?
Would she have lived longer because of these things?

As women in overdrive age, we remain active, busy, and
social. But just because we're aging differently and living longer doesn't mean we have to pass on the legacy of overwork,
inadequate rest, and lack of time for introspection. Women
can learn how to combat fatigue, say no, and become energized by passionate work and friendships. It's never too late
to understand the value of slowing down, relaxing, achieving
mindfulness, and meditating. And we can all educate ourselves
about the increasing number of readily available alternative
healing therapies.

This book will show you how. I'll talk about the things that
matter to women of all ages: how to fight fatigue through being
mindful and saying no; how to cultivate silence, slowness,
and relaxation amidst our busy lives. I'll discuss how to deal
with stresses both small and big in a positive way, and how to
approach longevity in every decade of your life. I'll also talk
about a holistic approach to aging in overdrive, explaining how
to address a variety of ailments with both Western and non-
Western medical approaches. I'll explore mind/body exercises
all women should know about. I'll discuss restoring the body

through sickness and disease and the role hormones play in our lives. Finally, I'll offer strategies about how to shift out of overdrive once and for all.

I find the current change in consciousness an exciting one. The more we clamor for change, the more these changes will affect the entire population for decades to come. The beauty of it is that we all gain in the end. It's thrilling to soak in the example of our mothers, colleagues, and friends so that we can all benefit from living longer, richer, and more fully embodied lives. It *is* possible to get out of overdrive and still live fulfilling and gratifying lives. So take a deep breath and discover what really matters.

—Nora Isaacs

combating low energy: brain drain and body blues

As I write this book, I am pregnant with my first child. And I'm tired. Every day, I sleep until nine-thirty, an hour when I'd have been showered, dressed, and comfortably settled at my computer with a cup of tea just a few short months ago. When three o'clock rolls around, I take a nap. I embrace the fact that pregnancy can be exhausting, and it makes sense: Transforming a bundle of cells into a human being takes a lot of energy. "Fatigue is also something that goes with the territory of being a woman," writes Patricia Fisher, author of *Age Erasers for Women*.[1] "Pregnancy and childbirth . . . devour enormous sums of energy." Understandable. But what I read next throws me into a state of panic. "So do the mood swings, headaches, diarrhea, and hot flashes that some women experience with the hormonal changes of menstruation, premenstrual syndrome, or menopause."

I see my future flash before my eyes. Is my newfound fatigue just a harbinger of the upcoming decades? Is this the beginning of decades of exhaustion that will effectively deplete my body of its hard-earned foundation of health? Maybe the situation is not *that* extreme, but I have to admit that I am girding myself for the months and the years to follow. As an overachieving woman who puts forth 100 percent effort at everything, whether it's work or play, how will I avoid burnout as my responsibilities increase? And how will I switch gears from the rigors of mothering as I move into my forties, fifties, and beyond? In the hyperaware state that is premotherhood, I've been searching for clues from women who've been there before me.

The Energetic Stages

In my twenties, I worked at a high-stress publishing job in Manhattan. I logged long hours, went to the gym after work, and then met friends for cocktails and late-night dinners. I didn't realize how far out of balance my life had become until I started having panic attacks. Needing to understand these sudden heart palpitations, choking sensations, and sweaty palms, I started going to therapy to talk about what might be behind the symptoms. There, I tried to unravel the feelings that accompanied my transition from student to full-time adult: individuating from my parents, living alone in a big city, and working and partying with equal intensity. By age twenty-four, I had experienced an exhaustion and burnout that women everywhere feel at various points in their lives. I recognized the signs of overdrive and knew that I was burning the candle at both ends. After some serious soul-searching, I realized I wanted to veer off the path I found myself on. I looked at my superiors—editors who still worked long hours and lived unbalanced lives thirty years after starting their careers. I didn't want my life to become a series of promotions that felt meaningless and empty; I yearned for a richness and vibrancy that I couldn't foresee myself experiencing in my current state. I knew I couldn't stay in Manhattan, so I did what so many people have done before me: I moved to California to start a new and more quiet life.

Not everyone has a burnout experience so early; for some, the big drain doesn't come until they experience motherhood. "Being a mother has been the most extraordinary experience of my life, and I wouldn't trade it for anything," writes Jan Hanson, L.Ac, in her book *Mother Nurture.*[2] "But by the time our son was three and his baby sister was a few months old, I had been working hard and living with stress for so long with so little replenishment that it all caught up with me. I kept going every day, but I had become very drained, both physically and emotionally. I saw variations on the same theme with my friends who were mothers. Some, like me, had hit bottom. Others felt their health and well-being were deteriorating, though some reserves remained inside. Many were still sailing along, yet even they were frazzled and tired."

This condition, which Hanson defines as "depleted mother syndrome," sets the stage for the next phase of a woman's life. When children are young, many women operate in "survival" mode. Waking up to feed the baby takes its toll after a while. Once the infant stage passes, the late nights get fewer, but the enormous energy output doesn't end. Running after a curious toddler rivals doing even the most strenuous workout. As children get older, superscheduled kids have rehearsals, practice, and social gatherings. When they become teenagers, the emotional toll on a parent may outweigh the physical output. Shuffling motherhood and a career takes thought and planning, but life for women without kids isn't any less strenuous. Women who also work full-time outside the home, travel, commute, and keep up their relationships have a full plate.

Living with depleted energy for years without end can result in high-grade levels of chronic stress; drained nutrients like vitamins, minerals, essential fatty acids, and amino acids; deregulated nervous, endocrine, or immune systems; and sometimes depression that won't go away.[3] By the time we reach our forties and fifties, sometimes we are so accustomed to fatigue, low energy, and exhaustion that our bodies simply don't know any other way of being.

But rather than simply losing a zest for living and zoning out mentally and physically, women today have an entire smorgasbord of possibilities and information available to combat residual fatigue from years past and counter any fatigue that results from the present. Once women settle into their routines as mature adults, be it with or without children, with the focus on career, primary relationship, or family life (or maybe all three), the balancing act of how to prioritize and manage it all can become overbearing. In later life, as the prospect of mortality becomes a reality, women are looking inward, making lifestyle changes, and creating lives where they feel energized and excited rather than depleted. But why wait until this stage to start this process of introspection? As Boomers forge new ground and women in their sixties are looking and living as women in their forties and fifties did a generation ago, they are paving the way for today's Gen Xers, who are entering their thirties and forties with an expectant attitude toward vitality, long life, and a smooth transition into old age.

But rather than simply losing a zest

for living and zoning out mentally

and physically, women today have an

entire smorgasbord of possibilities and

information available to combat residual

fatigue from years past and counter any

fatigue that results from the present.

Once women settle into their

routines as mature adults, be it with

or without children, and the focus on

career, primary relationship, or family

life (or maybe all three), the balancing

act of how to prioritize and manage

it all can become overbearing.

Taking on Fatigue: The Counterattack

Redefine Success

Eager to soak up information from those who have trodden the path before me, I often ask my elders what advice they might give a woman like me, in her thirties, when they look back on their lives so far. Luckily for me, this hasn't been difficult to do. My mother and I live in the same city and share a close relationship. Because of this, I am drawn to the wisdom of older women, and for some reason they are drawn to me. On vacation, in my yoga classes, even on the street, I always seem to connect with women a few stages ahead of me. Because of my background as a journalist, I have cultivated the habit of asking them a lot of questions and listening intently to their answers. Even though I've been interviewing for years, I'm consistently amazed at how much I can learn from other people and how much personal information people will reveal, if asked the right questions. Women who seem on the outside to have lived ordinary lives often have the most fascinating and compelling stories to tell and advice to give. As a woman in overdrive, I'm drawn to ask other women about their experiences operating in that same mode.

Throughout my years collecting informal data from those older than I, I've noticed a few common themes. Consistently, they say that they wish they had taken the time to evaluate the meaning of success, had worked to understand what makes them truly happy, and had incorporated these values into everyday life at an earlier stage. They tell me they wish they had understood this fundamental concept at a younger age so they could have cultivated a deeper sense of meaning and joy without spending years toiling at a job they disliked, staying in an unhealthy relationship, or waiting until a tragedy jolted them out of their misguided perceptions.

Many women tell me that experiencing periods of high energy doesn't necessarily involve a major change in habits, visits to sleep specialists, or any outward physical changes. Sometimes fatigue simply comes from decades of chasing after a hollow idea of success. The fix? An attitude adjustment. This comes in the form of redefining the meaning of "success," especially if we've taken lifelong cues that reinforce an external idea of success—having a prestigious position, an expensive car, a summer home.

I learned this firsthand recently, when on a magazine assignment in Hawaii for a story on a luxury vacation destination for wealthy and successful people. My husband, Eric, and I stayed in a $1,400-a-night room, dined on lobster, wore cushy robes, and had the bed turned down every night by the attentive staff. We marveled at a lifestyle that we don't often get to peek into. "This is the life!" we told each other while eating massive chocolate-covered strawberries on our private oceanside deck.

However, the next day we heard about the darker side of this seemingly idyllic existence from Calley O'Neill, resident yoga teacher and founder of the resort's wellness program. O'Neill teaches classes six days a week to a clientele that's 85 percent female and mostly over forty, many of whom are frequent travelers who work in high-stress, high-salary, and prestigious jobs: "They come to me at the end of the medical line," she said, referring to the fact that many of her students suffer from debilitating stress-related health problems like back pain, migraines, and chronic fatigue and have traveled across the country to top specialists for help. "These people feel so finite. They feel like they have to get it *all* now—and that this is all they have."[4] Her classes help to shift these women's perspective. She teaches them how to breathe, how to sit in silence, and how to alter their attitudes to help them understand that they hold infinite stores of peace and wisdom within them, regardless of their status or circumstance.

Fifty-year-old MaryAnn Gray, a social psychologist who lives in West L.A., found herself a victim of her own goals. After getting her PhD at age thirty, she threw herself into her career ("I worked my ass off!" she says), married in her mid-thirties, and spent the next decade under "huge amounts of work pressure." In her forties, she started questioning the meaning of success. "I began to ask myself, *How much of myself goes into work? What kind of person do I want to be?"* Only after she started to address these questions and ease off her work schedule did Gray have the space and time to explore her Jewish roots, join a Reform temple, and get in touch with a sense of spirituality that she hadn't connected with before. "I can't say I had a dramatic epiphany, but I like being part of a religious community. I like having an expression of my spirituality," she says.[5]

It's not likely that MaryAnn Gray or the resort's annual visitors will quit their jobs and join an ashram. But they will undoubtedly pay more attention to what makes them "sick and tired"—ultimately giving them more time, energy, and vigor in their everyday lives.

Find Your Passion

Feeling listless and uninspired could signal depression. Or it might mean that we're simply not tapping into the creative force that is inherent in each of us. I find the definition of the word "creativity" to be frustratingly narrow: "Creativity" is a huge term, one that encompasses a large array of possibilities beyond putting on a beret and getting out the easel and water-colors. We can be creative as real estate agents, accountants, or waitresses. We can tap into our creativity by cooking colorful meals, designing our own business stationery, or organizing the junk drawer. A yoga teacher I study with tells his students to let our postures become an expression of our fullness and creativity. Whenever he says this, I expand my lungs, take up more space, sharpen my senses, and drop into the experience a little more deeply. It feels wonderful. Once we think of ourselves as fully creative and complete beings, the more likely we'll feel energized and enthusiastic and allow our life force to pulse through and reveal itself.

Many women in overdrive find that they veered off track somewhere between entering the workforce and striving to succeed. Raising a family, working full-time, running a house-hold, and caring for sick parents on top of managing a busy work schedule don't leave a lot of extra time for creative pursuits. But growing older does allow more space for women to get back to their creative roots. After a twenty-year hiatus spent raising two daughters, my mother returned to oil painting—a passion that she had explored in her twenties and early thirties. Not that she hasn't always allowed her creativity to shine through:

Ideas and Books for Creativity

Excavating the depths of our own creative nature takes time and a little practice. When we are faced with the demons of fear, procrastination, and lack of time, it's easy to forget about nurturing our creative spirit. But don't. Instead, think of pushing your limits, taking a chance, and silencing your inner critic. Here are a few of my favorite books to help you get started:

The Artist's Way: A Spiritual Path to Higher Creativity, by Julia Cameron

The Vein of Gold: A Journey to Your Creative Heart, by Julia Cameron

Writing Down the Bones, by Natalie Goldberg

The Well of Creativity, by Natalie Goldberg

Bird by Bird: Some Instructions on Writing and Life, by Anne Lamott

She is known in our family for stylishly dressing in unique color combinations and creating sumptuous meals that look as good as they taste. But in her early fifties, this wasn't enough.

The resurrection happened during menopause. "I just got this surge of wanting to be creative and do something in addition to work," she says. "I always liked it and wanted to try some new things. The children were raised, and I had more time." She enrolled in a painting class and became totally invigorated by the experience. "It energized me," she says. "I felt I was doing something artistic; I loved working with the paint. When I'm painting, hours go by and I don't realize it; I'm in a different zone." Today, her living room is filled with her creations— Asian-inspired designs, impressionistic pieces, and still lifes— and visitors often comment on how dazzling they are and how they transform the space.

This idea of creation is especially important for females. According to Hinduism, the name for this is Shakti—the female energy that gives birth to everything. This is the power of creation. While women my age, expecting children or nurturing relatively new relationships or careers, may put their Shakti-energy into the physical creation of a child or the ambition of getting ahead or planning their careers, women of my mother's generation, women in their sixties, seventies, and beyond, can direct their Shakti to create other things: a piece of art or an idea, for instance. We can learn from each other and see how this energy manifests in marvelous and unpredictable ways over the course of our lives.

The Story of Shakti

According to an ancient spiritual system known as Tantra, the creation of the universe is explained through the interplay of Shiva and Shakti. Shiva represents the male principles and Shakti represents the female. From a metaphysical point of view, together these two forces embody the union of all opposites — light/dark, active/passive, male/female — and Tantra says that the whole universe is created, penetrated, and sustained by these two forces. In Hindu mythology, Shakti — which means "power" — is a powerful goddess also known as Kali and Durga, who helps barren women conceive and helps to cure the sick.

Get Enough Sleep

Sleep deprived? You aren't alone. The primary cause of fatigue among women might be the most obvious one: not enough sleep, restless sleep, or insomnia.

Thanks to fluctuating hormones, women are at least 30 percent more likely to experience sleep disturbances than their male counterparts. The idea of a good night's sleep seems so elusive for women for many reasons. As a pregnant woman, I find a good night's rest hard to come by. Because the baby is pressing down on my bladder, I get up five to six times each night to go to the bathroom. And when that isn't keeping me up, my thoughts and fears often do. Everyone says all of this night-waking is just preparing me for what's to come: long nights with a newborn, waking up every few hours to feed and change diapers. Professional women, both with and without children, also tell me they have trouble sleeping. In our thirties, many of us are trying to "make it" in our careers, proving ourselves to our superiors, putting in long hours, and doing whatever else it takes.

> *Thanks to fluctuating hormones,*
>
> *women are at least 30% more likely*
>
> *to experience sleep disturbances*
>
> *than their male counterparts.*

Perimenopause and menopause add another layer of possible sleep problems: Hormone shifts, low progesterone and estrogen levels, and lowered melatonin production can all lead to waking up with hot flashes, night sweats, or the inability to fall back to sleep. Ninety percent of women who visit menopause clinics cite fatigue as a prominent symptom, and more than 75 percent complain of insomnia.[6]

On the other hand, we simply need less sleep as we age, says Robert Greene, MD, author of *Perfect Balance: Dr. Robert Greene's Breakthrough Program for Finding the Lifelong Hormonal Health You Deserve.* He explains it this way: A major part of sleep is dedicated to processing information, and since we've already stored a good, solid information base by the time we enter midlife and beyond—and are therefore learning less on a day-to-day basis—we simply don't need as much time for this process to happen. "A newborn baby sleeps for up to twenty hours each day," says Greene. "But at age four, she'll need about twelve hours. By age ten, she'll feel rested after about ten hours of sleep, and from there her need for sleep will decline gradually so that by the time she's eligible for Medicare, she'll need only about six hours."

No matter how many hours you need, a restful night's sleep is essential. Greene says that after seventeen hours without sleep, most people operate as if they have a blood alcohol level of 0.05 percent![7] Women who suffer from sleep disorders, whether due to experiencing stress, overextending themselves, or going through menopause, can benefit from some common-sense lifestyle changes: Avoid caffeine after three in the afternoon and limit yourself to one glass of wine at night. Even better, avoid alcohol altogether, if you can. Eat a light, low-protein dinner. Eat foods high in tryptophan: turkey, bananas, figs, dates, yogurt, tuna, and nut butter. Avoid fatty or spicy foods that could cause heartburn. Drink warm milk or take a nice, relaxing hot bath before bed. Sometimes a lack of calcium and magnesium will cause you to wake up and not be able to get back to sleep; try taking supplements of these nutrients. If you take naps, make sure they last for a maximum of thirty minutes. Exercise regularly, but make sure that it's early in the day. Wake up at the same time each day, and keep your bedroom nice and dark. Relax before going to bed. And if you find yourself up worrying, write down your worries before you lie down or keep a journal next to your bed so that if you do wake up, you'll be able to express your fears and then get some shut-eye.

After seventeen hours without sleep,

most people operate as if they have

a blood alcohol level of 0.05%!

When I have trouble falling asleep, or going back to sleep, I borrow a guided relaxation technique from the yoga tradition. In my favorite sleep-inducing exercise, you close your eyes and focus on your toes. Imagine that your toes relax and sink into the bed. Then move on to your ankles, imagining them totally relaxing and releasing. Continue this process with every part of your body, envisioning that part relaxing, tension sliding away and vanishing. You'll be amazed at how soothing this feels, and I bet that most days you'll be fast asleep before you reach the top of your head. Other techniques include deep breathing into the abdomen and exhaling so that the abdomen pulls in, which sends signals to the nervous system and tells it to relax. Some people find that imagery also helps. Imagine your favorite natural setting: a beach, a meadow, a forest knoll. Imagine the wind on your face, the smell of the sea. Putting yourself in this relaxing place often helps to break the nonsleep cycle and lets you get a good night's rest.

Move Your Body

Health-conscious people everywhere know that exercise is the key to maintaining a healthy weight and avoiding a whole host of health problems. And although inertia isn't always on our side, especially as we age, exercise holds the key to combating low energy. Of course, other lifestyle changes—particularly nutritional, which I'll discuss in Chapter 9—also play a major role, but exercise is really the cornerstone when it comes to aging. In fact, a MacArthur Foundation Study on Aging in America found that exercising regularly is the key to optimum aging (the other two are avoiding chronic diseases and staying engaged in meaningful relationships).[8]

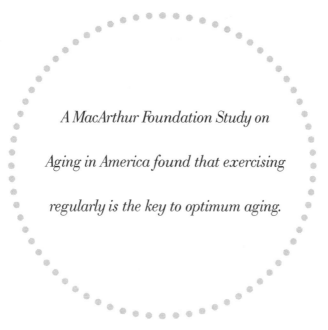

A MacArthur Foundation Study on

Aging in America found that exercising

regularly is the key to optimum aging.

"I actually enjoy physical exercise," says Terry Ferretti, a wife of forty years, mother of two daughters, and grandmother. "If I can do things physically, I know mentally I am going to feel better."[9] The conclusions of decades' worth of studies couldn't have articulated this better. And while research backs up Ferretti's statement, no amount of data adequately illustrates the feeling of fresh air against your skin after a day indoors, of the trajectory from low energy at the beginning of a run to that high feeling afterward, or of the exhilaration of jumping into a cold pool to swim laps.

And exercise doesn't have to be boring or routine. It can be an expression of joy and playfulness. Once Ferretti reached her fifties, she went back to a favorite exercise of hers: dancing. "It coordinates the mind and the muscles," she says. "I had the time of my life!" Not only did the movement help her physically, she says it helped her get through the grieving process after her sister died.

MaryAnn Gray attributes her high energy and, most recently, her "easy" menopause in part to her rigorous workout schedule. "I work out at the gym like a maniac!" she says. As part of her regimen, she works out "hard" with a trainer three times a week. "I keep pushing myself," she says, and that helps her to stay youthful. "I feel very healthy and energetic," she says. "Of course, I look older and I see visible signs of aging. My body will never look like the twenty- or thirty-year-olds'," she admits, quickly adding, "but I feel like I have gained a lot more confidence professionally and feel like I have gained some strength of character."

I asked my sister, Elana, about the role of exercise in her life. At thirty-seven, she's been doing one form or another of movement her whole life. She walks and hikes, but dance has always been her favorite form of exercise. She says the most important factor when it comes to exercise is that it be accessible. "I do any sort of exercise that feels authentic and fits into the flow of my day," she says. "I find that it's so much easier to do. It feels natural and not like a 'should,' which has always been important to me. When I *should* myself about exercise, then I don't do it." For Elana, the benefits are major. "I feel more expansive," she says. "It gets me out of my head and into my body and gives me a bigger sense of myself and the possibilities." It also has a significant impact on her breathing, since she says she's struggled with shallow breathing for much of her life. "It's a natural way of getting the flow of my breath back." When it comes down to it, exercise plays a key role in how my sister looks and feels: "The truth is," she says, "a lot of people are surprised at my age, but it has a lot to do with how much I move and dance. Dance is exercise, and it's also play and creative expression. Those things are really tied together for me. They are a part of what helps me feel and be young and not look my age."

Whether it's dancing, walking, doing yoga or tai chi, playing tennis, jogging, or working out with a trainer, staying physically active works: It can improve mood and relieve depression; prevent or delay some types of cancer, heart disease, and diabetes; and restore the 20 to 40 percent of strength and muscle tissue that we lose when we age, in a process known as sarcopenia.[10]

Exercise can improve mood and

relieve depression; prevent or delay

some types of cancer, heart disease,

and diabetes; and restore the

20–40% of strength and muscle

tissue we lose when we age, in a

process known as sarcopenia.

Of course, if you feel excessively tired for no apparent reason or experience muscle and joint pain, headaches, or difficulty concentrating or sleeping, you should see a doctor. Because there is no specific laboratory test or clinical sign for chronic fatigue syndrome (CFS), no one knows how many people are affected by this illness. The Centers for Disease Control and Prevention (CDC) estimates, however, that as many as 500,000 people in the United States have CFS or a CFS-like condition.[11]

The Centers for Disease Control and

Prevention estimates, however, that

as many as 500,000 people in the

United States have Chronic Fatigue

Syndrome or a CFS-like condition.

Chronic fatigue is three times more prevalent in women than in men; nine out of ten people who have fibromyalgia (a rheumatic disorder similar to CFS) are women. No one knows exactly what causes these illnesses; some attribute chronic fatigue to a virus that disrupts the immune and endocrine systems. A recent 2006 study reports that chronic fatigue might involve a genetic component that reduces people's ability to deal with stress.[17] Although the research is murky, strengthening the immune system through diet and exercise to restore low energy can only help. Women also say that acupuncture, homeopathic medicine, and vitamins and herbs seem to alleviate the symptoms. When you look at these illnesses with a holistic eye, it seems that finding ways to come back into balance, giving yourself time to relax, and rethinking your priorities could be an important part of your recovery.

Chronic fatigue is three times more prevalent in women than in men; 9 out of 10 people who have fibromyalgia (a rheumatic disorder similar to CFS) are women.

chapter 2

cultivating
slowness and
relaxation

Because of the incredible amount of energy consumed by
growing a baby, I am treating myself with the utmost respect
to make sure that I assist my body in the work it needs to do.
I've stepped up the way I care for myself: I sleep until I wake
up naturally, instead of setting the alarm. I eat healthy foods
and incorporate several small meals a day instead of three large
ones. I exercise moderately, just a little every day. When stressful thoughts arise, as they inevitably do, I put them into a larger
perspective and let them go. Most of all, I'm slowing down in
the hopes of restoring my body and mind in preparation for the
hectic period that will surely follow.

Training myself to return to a slower state of mind, I'm discovering, requires rigorous discipline. I have to be unrelentingly
vigilant. Checking email while on the phone? Unacceptable.
Running into the kitchen during a commercial break to chop
veggies? A no-no. I have replaced my habit of bolting out of bed
when the alarm sounds with five deep breaths and a sweet hello
to my baby. Instead of merging with the forward-moving mass
on the underground train, I move off to the side, repeating

the words *Slow down*. I now leave for appointments a half hour early, waving on aggressive motorists and walking around the block for no apparent reason.

Small changes, admittedly, but I was shocked at how much effort and awareness even these took. Realizing that my time alone is now finite and my days of relative leisure might end soon, I have retrained myself to slow down—to soak up every moment.

Growing another human being is a massive responsibility, and I want to get it right. But lately I've started to wonder: Why did it take having an unborn child's health to worry about for me to become aware of slowing down? Why does caring for others take priority over caring for ourselves? Why don't we set up our lives so that we get enough sleep, eat well, exercise, slow down, and give ourselves the space to be imperfect?

The energy spent on negative or obsessive thinking could be much better spent contributing something to your friends, family, and the world.

Pregnancy hasn't always been a time to slow down, turn down obligations, and reflect on where we were headed. Women like sixty-one-year-old Terry Ferretti told me about the attitudes in the seventies, when she was pregnant and raising small children. "In those days they didn't say, 'It's okay to be selfish—take time for yourself,'" she says. "No, you came last!" she recalls. For my generation, I feel that the pendulum has swung slightly to a more balanced position. It's more socially acceptable to "take time for yourself," as Ferretti puts it.

But I realize that I have internalized that feeling of "needing to do it all"—even though the outside pressure isn't as great. It's the pressure I put on myself. A nagging voice disrupts my thoughts if I sleep in late or leave dishes in the sink: *You're lazy. You're not working hard enough. You're not contributing enough to your relationship.* The most interesting part of this whole exercise has been being in tune with my thoughts: the guilt at feeling "lazy," the self-judgment when I'm not as productive as usual, and the negative feelings when I'm not a "perfect" person. Most women, whether they are single or married, old or young, can relate to these nagging thoughts. I know that these free-floating thoughts probably do more harm than the "harmful" action itself. Physically, I believe that most disease comes from a feeling of "dis-ease," or not feeling easeful and peaceful in the world. Mentally, the energy spent on negative or obsessive thinking could be much better spent contributing positive energy to your friends, family, and the world.

A nagging voice disrupts my thoughts

if I sleep in too late or leave dishes in

the sink: You're lazy. You're not working

hard enough. You're not contributing

enough to your relationship.

Although my parents taught me that outward accomplishments aren't the highest goals to aspire to, the pesky notion that maybe they really *are* is deeply ingrained by our societal values that orient us toward material success. Once we start running on overdrive, it's hard to get off. And we certainly don't get any help from society, which praises "accomplishment," frowns upon slowing down as "lazy," and expects women to perform at high levels of efficiency for extended periods of time. That elicits the question: When very real obligations exist, how do we, as women, reconcile this with the need to get a little rest? In other words, how do we turn down the heat?

The Slow Movement

As we age, our bodies need less stimulation and more silence. Carl Honoré's book *In Praise of Slowness* spawned the Slow Movement, an informal collection of groups and individuals who believe in the premise that "we can live better if we live more slowly." According to Honoré, the idea for the book came to him after he toyed with the idea of buying a book of one-minute bedtime stories for his son. "Suddenly it hit me," he writes. "My rushaholism has gotten so out of hand that I'm even willing to speed up those precious moments with my son at the end of the day. *There has to be a better way,* I thought, because living in fast-forward is not really living at all."[1] After he began investigating, Honoré realized what a huge toll speed is taking on our lives: The quality of our work, health, and relationships suffers drastically because we move so fast. The sad fact is that statistics show that on average, American adults now work fifty hours per week, up nine hours from the 1970s, when people reported working only forty-one hours a week.[2]

> *Statistics show that on average*
>
> *American adults now work 50*
>
> *hours per week, up 9 hours from*
>
> *the 1970s, when people reported*
>
> *working only 41 hours a week.*
>
> **Source: Harris Interactive:**
> **www.harrisinteractive.com/harris_poll/**

After reading Honoré's book, I began to cultivate my own personal Slow Movement, which has been a gradual move toward greater self-awareness and patience with myself. I have been working on this self-improvement project since I left my publishing job in New York City eight years ago. Little by little, I have learned that although slower isn't always better, it helps to frame my life in this way. Rather than just charging forward, the concept of slowness tells me to be conscious of what I'm doing. In the end, I might still choose speed—but at least I've slowed down enough to make that choice. As we age, we can draw from our own wisdom and be cognizant of this choice, over and over again.

Moving fast doesn't just happen by driving fast down the highway or rushing from one errand to the next. It is the constant inundation with information that comes at us at warp speed from every direction. As I've gotten older, I've realized how the speed of information affects me. I read more magazines than books (it's faster!). I check my email twenty times a day, whereas only a few years back I might have checked once or twice (someone might need me!). I drive to places I could just as easily walk to (why waste the time?). I am reachable via cell phone all of the time (there may be an emergency!). The so-called advances of our time are really just another example of out-of-control speed.

In my last apartment we had cable TV because it came with the unit. I'd never had cable, and over the months I realized that I was watching more and more. When I felt bored. When I didn't feel like working. When I felt as if I needed background noise. Then I started to feel the pull toward the television. I became involved in the soap opera of celebrity lives. I began planning my workday around *Oprah*. Even though I was going nowhere, I had become addicted to the fast-moving images on the screen, the excitement of the lifestyles of the rich and famous, and the idea that I had to fill my time with noise and motion and activity. This had to stop. When we moved we decided not to get cable; we even opted out of the basic stations. It was only then that I realized the negative effects of so much technology on my life. Instead of savoring my quiet time and enjoying my solitude, I immediately filled it. Part of slowness, I discovered, is allowing the space for stillness.

Take It Down a Notch

With all of the very real demands on our time, how do we take it down a notch? I asked this question of busy women like forty-one-year-old Keren Taylor, executive director of WriteGirl, a creative writing and mentoring program for girls, who labels herself a workaholic.[3] Keren is one of four million self-employed women in America, representing nearly 6 percent of all employed women.[4] She is responsible for the inner workings of this nonprofit, which she runs out of her home. She is driven, ambitious, passionate—and busy. "If I have a goal, I want to make it happen," she says. But recently, after going through early menopause, she had to slow down and think about her life. Because of her very physical reminder of aging, she says she's started to look at the "big picture." This includes taking time away from her business, where she could potentially work all day and all night. Recently, Keren made the decision to have a 6 PM cutoff time. She has had to make it part of her routine to stop working to allow herself to take it down a notch.

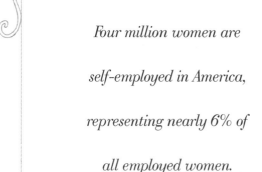

Four million women are

self-employed in America,

representing nearly 6% of

all employed women.

Source: U.S. Department of Labor:
www.dol.gov/wb/stats/main.htm

When six o'clock rolls around, no matter what she's involved with, she leaves her desk and everything that has gone undone. She's also started going for hikes without her cell phone, another major shift in her routine.

Keren also tries to integrate stress-reduction techniques that don't feel too overwhelming to her schedule. For example, the idea of spending a day at a spa always sounded like a luxury she couldn't afford in terms of the time commitment, so she never scheduled massages before. But recently, she found a massage center close to her house; she knows that she can enjoy a forty-five-minute massage without giving up her day. "There's no showers or saunas, but it's dreamy that it's so close to home," she says.

Keren says it's also become crucial for her to plan vacations well in advance: "Those are blackout dates where I can let go; I know the work is finite—otherwise it becomes infinite and I don't get a respite."

But even vacations can be stressful. Beyond the planning and decision-making, there is the hidden danger of *thinking* we're slowing down without really slowing down. Consider what it takes to plan a vacation. Beyond the research, calls, and emails, a "stress-busting" vacation often involves a frenzied week before you leave to get everything done. Not to mention that in order to pay for a vacation, some people have to work overtime or be stressed about finances!

Like many urban folks, I love living in a city partly because of the options: great restaurants, nonstop entertainment, new art openings every night. Evenings and weekends fill up with fun things to do, friends to meet, visitors to entertain. Although these activities feed the spirit in one way, they have the potential to deplete it in another. During an interview with Juliet Schor, the wonderful author of *The Overworked American: The Unexpected Decline of Leisure* and *The Overspent American: Why We Want What We Don't Need,* we discussed the reasons for this push and pull. Although the time we spend engaging in things that are emotionally and intellectually fulfilling can feel like a luxury, these are often still very structured activities, technically not the same as time off or unstructured downtime. According to Schor, unstructured time holds the key to true slowness. Whether it's a vacation or a night out, even the fun things in life still require scheduling, planning, and taking action. It's the unstructured time that leaves us refreshed and rejuvenated. It's

those treasured days when we find nothing on our daily planners that allow for true rest: lounging around the house, playing with children or pets, having a spontaneous phone call with
an old friend.

It's the unstructured time that leaves

us refreshed and rejuvenated. It's those

treasured days when we find nothing on

our daily planners that allow for true rest:

lounging around the house, playing with

children or pets, having a spontaneous

phone call with an old friend.

This leisure time isn't just a luxury. According to doctors, it's *essential* to staying young. If you don't get enough leisure time in your life, you'll feel grouchy and tired. Over time, life without leisure can lead to more serious health problems, like heart disease, ulcers, and high blood pressure.[5] Yet, for many women, this idea of unstructured time has fallen by the wayside. I notice that even when I have a free morning, or in rare cases a full free day, I have to fight the urge to make a to-do list or fill up the time with things that don't really need doing at that very moment. I'm programmed to accomplish a certain amount in a given day. One more thing to cross off the list, one more thing to offer a sense of completion. Before I realize what's happening, I start treating my leisure time like a job! Experts say the key is to replace this task-oriented approach with a feeling of playfulness and fun.[6] But my life isn't set up for that. Just when I finish one thing, another begins. Just when I think I've put something behind me, it's back again. Stopping this cycle takes constant self-monitoring, but it's worth it.

Slow Down: Walking Meditation

Learn to slow down with this simple yet challenging form of meditation. Find an area where you can walk: It's nice to do this outside, but if that's not possible, you can just walk around the perimeter of a room. Have your hands at your sides. Start by walking slowly and deliberately, without any particular destination. Breathe naturally and deeply into your belly so that your focus is on your inhalations and exhalations. Once you fall into that rhythm, bring one hand to your abdomen and the other hand on top of the first hand. Look down at the ground about three feet in front of you. Start to coordinate your movement with your breath: On an inhalation, slowly raise the heel of the right foot, leaning slightly forward to maintain your balance. With the foot lifted and toes touching the ground, exhale. On an inhalation, raise your right foot off the ground and bring it forward. On an exhalation, drop your right foot to the floor. Think about each of the movements as you are doing them: lifting, raising, shifting, dropping. Do this to the left side. After about twenty minutes of this movement, release your hands to the side. Continue to observe your breath for another minute, and then finish the meditation with any peaceful thought that you like.

Voluntary Simplicity

Another movement I've been watching over the years, one that stresses quality over quantity, is called voluntary simplicity. Popularized with the books *Voluntary Simplicity: Toward a Way of Life That Is Outwardly Simple, Inwardly Rich,* and *Your Money or Your Life,* the trend centers on the idea that much of our speed has to do with a race for material possessions—and all it takes to obtain them, keep them, and get more.

"We can describe voluntary simplicity as a manner of living that is outwardly more simple and inwardly more rich, a way of being in which our most authentic and alive self is brought into direct and conscious contact with living," writes *Voluntary Simplicity* author Duane Elgin. "This way of life is not a static condition to be achieved but an ever-changing balance that must be continuously and consciously made real."[7]

Once the desire for these items is diminished, the thinking goes, we have room to create slower and simpler lives, whether that means retiring earlier, working less, or just taking up hobbies that we love but keep putting off. Getting off the spending treadmill requires a brutal examination of how we spend our money, and ultimately making choices to do without certain conveniences that might actually be preventing us from living life to its fullest.

"To live more simply is to unburden ourselves—to live more lightly, cleanly, aerodynamically. It is to establish a more direct, unpretentious, and unencumbered relationship with all aspects of our lives: the things we consume, the work that we do, our relationships with others, our connections with nature and the cosmos, and more. Simplicity of living means meeting life face-to-face."[8]

How to live on less than you think you can? It takes some sacrifice. If your mortgage is more than you can handle, rent instead of buy. Buy used furniture and clothing instead of new. Sell your car and take public transportation. Ditch your cell phone and your cable TV. Make your morning cup of coffee at home instead of spending $2.50 on a latte. Pack your lunch instead of buying it. Get rid of your credit cards, or use them with discretion: A friend once told me that she put her credit cards in a cup of water and froze them, forcing herself to really have to plan ahead when using her credit card instead of spending impulsively.

For me, this begins with challenging my assumptions and priorities. As a new parent, I want to teach my child values that highlight spirit over substance. But I realize I have to live these values first. Growing up, my sister and I had our own rooms. I admit I liked the privacy. My husband, on the other hand, shared a room with two of his cousins. I had always assumed that sharing a room represented a hardship and that he always longed for his own room. I had placed judgments on these things: Big room is good, shared room is bad. But this wasn't so. He loved the closeness and the company of sharing a room; to this day he feels a special bond with those cousins. So the key is to look at the judgments we place on our lives and ask ourselves with brutal honesty: What do we *really* need to live a happy life?

Hurry Up and Slow Down

For Keren Taylor, slowing down happened by accident. She says that she couldn't ignore the signs of aging when her hot flashes started at forty-one years old. The confusing part, she says, is that she looks young and feels even younger. Thus, she's confronted with the difficult emotional and spiritual effects of aging earlier than most other women. As a busy working woman, she's had to explore what kinds of things help her cope with this sudden onslaught of symptoms. I asked her if she's found anything that works. "Going deeper into the things that I love," she replied. What a beautiful sentiment. She spoke about abandoning her preoccupation with counting calories and losing weight, spending more time with her dog in the woods, and indulging herself in the times she's not working instead of incessant thoughts that tell her she "should" be working. Most important, perhaps, was abandoning the notion of worrying about what other people think. "When you are in a public field, head of an organization like I am, it's easy to get caught up in these thoughts: *Do they like me? Was I too abrupt?* I'm trying to let go of that. If it comes from a true place of wanting to be passionate and true and move things forward, then it doesn't matter."

Simple Ways to Slow Down

Turn off the television.

Plan one fewer activity a week.

Eat dinner as a family.

Find a quiet hobby, like knitting, gardening, or walking.

Leave enough time to get places so you don't have to rush. If you do have to rush, breathe deeply while you do it.

Take a two- to five-minute mini-meditation in the middle of the day: Stop what you are doing and sit there.

Breathe. Smile.

Slowing down must come from an internal place. As working women, we can blame our bosses and our jobs, but Keren's situation proves that ultimately it's our responsibility. Because she owns her own business, she creates her own stress level. As her own boss, she can see the direct results of her failures and successes. "Not meeting the company's goals," she says, "means not meeting the goals that I've set. That's even more stressful than working for The Man. If you fail, you feel the direct results of your failure. In a company you get a second chance." For Keren and other self-employed women, overdrive is hard to escape—but not impossible.

The truth is that most of us work for someone else. If you work for others, it's important to check in with yourself several times a day. If you feel lethargic, take a walk. If you have committed to a lunch date with a coworker but need alone time, ask to reschedule. When it's time to leave for the day, commit to leaving. Part of women's desire to please extends to the workplace. But we don't have to put in "face time" to please our superiors. It's our choice to have balance.

Part of women's desire to please extends to the workplace. But we don't have to put in "face time" to please our superiors. It's our choice to have balance.

Hidden Moments and Meditation

Many women can't slow down. We might have young children and older parents to take care of. Maybe we need to work two jobs. Don't despair; slowing down isn't impossible for anyone. Taking a few hidden moments throughout the day can help women remember to slow down, if even for a moment.

I encourage my yoga students to start the day slowly, resist the temptation to go into "doing" mode right away. I have to fight the urge to check my email or make a phone call to New York. The key is to bring ourselves back to the mantra *Slow down*. I know mornings can be hectic, and many people balk at the idea of spending twenty minutes doing anything but getting ready. I tell them to do something quiet instead of bolting out of bed and starting in with the craziness of the day. Personally, I've done many things over the years. One is to wake up and set a clear intention for the day: What do I want to accomplish? I then think about some manageable goals I set for myself. This isn't just a to-do list, and might include something like Eat a Healthy Lunch or Respond to a Friend with Compassion Instead of Judgment. What do I want to let go of? I then think of certain behaviors and habits that aren't serving me. This could include a growing feeling of regret over something that already passed or a feeling of inadequacy because of my own internal negative thinking. Because I've spent so many years with my yoga practice, I am personally fond of the loving-kindness meditation: "May all beings be happy/May all beings be well/May all beings be peaceful and at ease."

chapter 3

squelching stress and elevating the spirit

My father often reminds me of the time I called him up from college. "Dad," I asked him, "how do you get spiritual?" He laughed when I asked him this, but the yearning behind the question was real. I knew I wanted more than a perfectly mediocre life, and finding a way to become more spiritual seemed to me the logical way to achieve something more meaningful.

Going through the trials and angst of my twenties, I felt I needed something to ground me and get me through the challenges of that time: Experiencing heartbreak, changing friendships, finding a first job, moving to a big city, and taking on the responsibility of becoming an adult created stress for an overachieving, people-pleasing person like myself. I wanted to find ways to learn to cope with these big changes gracefully, rather than rely on the ways I saw around me: drugs, alcohol, and unhealthy relationships, among the most popular.

This yearning to "get spiritual" exists within all of us. But when we operate in overdrive and a state of being overwhelmed, sometimes it seems as if connecting with this essence is our last priority. The state of overdrive is by no means a "women's problem," but with women taking on so many roles in today's culture, the chances are likely that these roles will at some point clash, leaving us burned out and stressed to the max. Over time, unrelieved stress can lead to serious stress-related disorders, including fatigue, insomnia, depression, reduced immune functioning, and low libido. Ironically, if we can understand how hooking into a sense of spirituality could help us deal with stress, more women might actually take the time out to cultivate this part of ourselves.

When life's everyday problems arise—our bosses yell at us, our partners instigate a fight, our children push us over the edge—we learn to deal with stress in that moment. But what about the stress resulting from major life changes that inevitably arise in our adult lives—dealing with the death of a parent, going through a divorce, or taking care of elderly parents—and whose effects linger far longer than a fight with our spouse? And how do we find a sense of spirit within these dramatic and often traumatic events in our lives? Many of us wait until one of these traumatic or life-altering moments happens to connect with spirituality. But if we wait to call upon our spirituality when going through hard times, how can we access it if we're out of practice?

The state of overdrive is by no means

a "woman's problem," but with women

taking on so many roles in today's culture,

the chances are likely that these roles

will at some point clash, leaving us

burned out and stressed to the max.

Women of all ages tell me that taking care of young children is the first of many major long periods of intense stress they experienced, testing boundaries and changing the course of a life. Each subsequent decade and every big change, planned and unplanned, often brings with it a new stressful event that requires us to mobilize our strength to deal with what lies ahead. For many of us, this means calling on our sense of spirituality to get us through—or discovering our own inner wisdom that we didn't even know we had.

Those who have been through high-stress events have talked to me about how they dealt with the most stressful situations in their lives. No matter what their specific situation, it was remarkable how these women all described a very similar trajectory when it comes to stress and the spirit. In very similar language, they all described a feeling of "losing themselves" or "not knowing who they were." As time went on, they began to see their experience as an opportunity for growth and awakening of the spirit. Forty-one-year-old Sarah Nesson, whose father died suddenly of a heart attack at the age of sixty-six, explained this notion beautifully:

> *You have to lose yourself to find yourself more deeply than you ever have before. I used to think a lot that having a spiritual life meant that things feel good, or that having contact with God makes you feel better. I still fall into that from time to time, but what I really learned from losing someone who meant so much to me is that it's part of a journey and part of making contact with God. To go deeply into the darkness, the unknown, and the grief, and let myself feel very young and very scared made me a more whole person. I have carried that wisdom with me, and now when*

I see difficult times coming, I feel more willing to be in touch with that part of myself. I seem to be so much stronger. I assume if there is another major stressor in my life, I can just hang on. I would trade back having my father in a second; however, I am also grateful for all that's happened, psychologically and spiritually. I'm a more compassionate, wiser, and deeper soul. I'm grateful for what I've gained.

Sarah's Story: Dealing with Loss

Sarah Nesson, now a graduate student, says that the day her father died suddenly of a heart attack sent her life into a tailspin for years to come. Her father was a beloved doctor and hospital administrator, and a thousand people showed up at his funeral. For the first few months after his death, Sarah and her family stayed busy learning the details of his life and all of the people he'd affected. The letters and calls never stopped coming, and Sarah felt intensely proud of her father and his achievements. A few months later, when Thanksgiving came around, however, Sarah started to get depressed.

"Thanksgiving just did me in," she says. "It was the worst Thanksgiving I've ever known." She fell into a deep depression, with the classic symptoms: She wasn't eating or sleeping well; she experienced periods of high anxiety; and her ambitions to become a rabbi faded to the background.

Sarah took the opportunity to draw on her sense of spirituality that she had cultivated since her teen years; she already had a yoga, meditation, and Buddhist practice. At the time her father passed away, she was working on a play with a traveling Jewish theater about Shabbat and had been going to Friday-night services for a few years.

"I was extremely grateful that I had a spiritual practice to draw on," she says. "But in those months of devastation, there wasn't much that I was able to do that was very comforting." One day in December still stands out in her mind. Still deeply depressed, she mustered up the courage to prepare her house for Sabbath, lighting candles, making a fire, and cleaning the house. "I don't even think I sang the blessing, but I just remember how vivid it looked after I lit the candles and saying this small prayer of gratitude and seeing how beautiful it was. It was a sense of homecoming. To return to a practice when things are really, really dark like that takes courage and fortitude."

She also found that the creative process helped with her high stress levels and connected her to her spirit. A classical pianist, she began to write songs, including three about losing her dad. She also planned a concert called "Leap of Faith," which she dedicated to her father. "It was tremendously valuable to have music to share about my journey, my relationship, the different colors, playing piano, and being able to express myself that way. I consider that my spiritual practice."

Creating some space around her also immensely helped. After reading a book that suggested taking some time every day to just "be," she started setting aside a little time for herself, whether it was getting under a blanket on the couch, sitting with her father's photo, or going for walks every morning near a lake and just sitting and watching the ducks. Close girlfriends who had both lost their mothers as young women also helped her through that winter. "For the first time in my adult life, I really let my friends know just how frightened, lost, and depressed I felt," she says.

After many months, the light soon revealed itself to her. Through her rituals, religion, friends, and therapist, she says she began to "claw myself out from under darkness. I built a stronger sense of myself than I ever had. It was an incredible rite of passage." She explains it this way: "In shamanic terms, a crisis like the ones we're talking about is called dismemberment: a necessary taking apart of yourself so you can put yourself back together in a deeper way—and that's the gift of dismemberment."

I thought about Sarah's words for a long time. I loved the visual image of dismemberment: the idea of putting the pieces of a puzzle back together, but so it's more stable than it was before. Her words helped me to understand what women go through when they lose someone they love. She was not only dealing with the loss of her father, but also with the complicated father-daughter relationship that most of us have with our fathers, seeking their approval, seeing them both as all too human and at the same time objects of adoration. Sarah's fortitude inspired me to keep on cultivating my own spiritual life through spending time with friends, being creative, and diving deeply into pain rather than avoiding it.

Jackie's Story: The Pain of Divorce[1]

People age forty and older generally feel that divorce is more emotionally devastating than job loss, about equal to experiencing a major illness, and nearly as devastating as a spouse's death, according to a survey conducted for *AARP The Magazine* called "The Divorce Experience: A Study of Divorce at Midlife and Beyond." The same study found that 66 percent of women claimed to have initiated their split, which disputes many long-held assumptions about mid- and late-life divorce.[2] But for fifty-four-year-old Jackie Overton, this wasn't the case. After more than twenty years of marriage, her husband left her for another woman. With three kids, ages twenty-one, nineteen, and sixteen, Jackie says she has been in constant overdrive mode since the divorce. Handling financial worries, having disputes with her husband's lawyers, caring for her children, and dealing with her anger have all caused her an intense amount of stress.

After the traumatic event, Jackie recalls walking around overcome with anger. She took comfort in the things that grounded her: reading books, praying, and going to therapy. To help deal with the stress, she did meditation, chanting, and yoga and talked to a higher power. "I try to ask God to help me deal with my kids; they are challenging right now. I work really hard and want to have a life still, but I want to be there for my kids. It takes some balancing and I have some guilt. I try to do everything, but I also need to be kind to myself."

People age 40 or older generally

feel that divorce is more emotionally

devastating than losing a job, about

equal to experiencing a major

illness, and nearly as devastating as

a spouse's death. The same study

found that 66% of women claimed

to have initiated their split, which

disputes many long-held assumptions

about mid- and late-life divorce.

Source: *AARP The Magazine*

Jackie also found a passion: swing-dancing lessons. "I fell in love, and I use swing dancing as medication, an antidepressant." Her husband didn't like to dance, so Jackie hadn't really let loose in more than two decades. Now she looks forward to her classes and also finds that they're a great way to meet people. Her supportive family and network of friends shepherded her through her darkest days. Despite the help from others around her, however, she knew that she had to take responsibility for herself and her future. She made an effort to make some single friends in addition to her married ones. She kept a positive attitude. She went to singles events, even if she had to go by herself. "Sometimes I just didn't want to go, but I always ended up having a good time." Every day she wakes up and looks for something good to feel grateful for.

Although the divorce continues to be stressful, Jackie says she turned a corner when she could start to see the benefits of the traumatic event. The divorce helped her face reality. "After I realized that he was seeing someone else, I realized just how bad my marriage was and how I had buried that. I ended up thanking God for helping me out of a bad situation." She's lost more than forty pounds on her five-foot, five-inch frame. "I was so unhappy in my marriage that I ate for emotional comfort," she says. "After he left, I realized I didn't need to derive comfort from food."

She found her spiritual core strong and steady, and she called on it every single day. "I never was angry at God—I don't believe God is that kind of god." Instead, she adopted the ideas of the Buddha, who said that suffering comes when we try to keep things status quo and get attached to them. "If you attach

to this you will suffer more," she says. "Letting go of my identity as a wife, or a mother, was painful, but I saw there was an
opportunity. After getting through the initial part, and being so
totally shaken up, I realized that I could do it."

The ramifications of the divorce are far from over. Jackie still
must deal with lawyers and figure out finances. She has to learn
to date all over again and make the decision about whether to
stick with her husband's surname or change it back. She must
deal with the fallout of the divorce on her three children.

As someone who just celebrated her two-year wedding
anniversary, I asked Jackie for some parting advice about love.
What could her experience teach me, someone just starting
out on the path?

"Keep working on the marriage; don't let it get so distant that there's nothing left—and that can happen," she said.
"Women have a lot of power when it comes to relationships.
Men are really simple creatures—they really are. Learn how
to ask for things you want; learn how to give and take. Have
fun in the relationship. When you stop having fun, it will slide
downhill." When it comes to dealing with stress, Jackie had
one word for me: exercise. "It's the most powerful thing,
mentally and physically. Everyone thinks I look ten years
younger." When she started exercising, she says, her
cholesterol and triglycerides dropped, her asthma improved,
and her elevated pulse rate decreased. "You've got to find what
you love to do, like I found dancing and yoga," she says. "And
once you do, keep doing it."

Ronnie's Story: Older Motherhood

Like so many other stereotypes that don't hold true anymore, neither does that of the new mom in her twenties and thirties experiencing the birth of her first child. The trend of older women having babies continues to increase over time. From 2003 to 2004, the birth rate for women age thirty to thirty-four increased by about 1 percent; the birth rate for women age thirty-five to thirty-nine rose by 4 percent; and the birth rate for women age forty to forty-five increased 3 percent.[3] With the marriage delay, multiple families, and advances in fertility treatments, older motherhood is becoming more commonplace than ever. But that doesn't mean it's easy. Becoming an "older mother" brings its own set of challenges. Physically, women who've been through pregnancy in their forties find it harder on their bodies; many feel more fatigued than their twenty-year-old counterparts.

Ronnie Ruggies, a therapist living in New Jersey, became unexpectedly pregnant at the age of forty-five. Now fifty-seven with a twelve-year-old son, Ruggies says the stresses of being an older mom—and all of the emotional and practical issues that come with it—are impossible even to put into words. "Most of the other mothers are younger than I am, and I just can't keep up with them," she says. "Most of them are wealthy and not working," she adds. Ruggies still maintains her full-time job to help with the family finances and finds herself completely isolated from other women—and sometimes from herself. "There is a shift in consciousness that comes with this age," she says. "My husband is sixty, and we are battling being parents."

In 2002, birth rates for women age

35 to 39 and age 40 to 44 were the

highest in more than 30 years—

41 births per 1,000 women and 8

per 1,000 women, respectively. From

1990 to 2002, the number of babies

born to women age 40 to 44 nearly

doubled—from 48,607 to 95,788.

Source: The National Center for Health
Statistics, part of the federal Centers for
Disease Control and Prevention

Ruggies, who considered herself a hippie at one point, says she's lost touch with that sense of freedom and openness that defined her being. Now, she says, she struggles with the fact that she "doesn't know who she is." Between the full-time parenting, working, and running the household, she longs for the days when she thought about herself and her needs.

Ronnie's story is one side of the coin when it comes to women having babies later in life. On the other side are women in their forties who are desperate to get pregnant. The stress experienced from infertility can undo many women, both emotionally and financially. The other options, surrogate parenting and adoption, can cause great amounts of angst and take an immense toll on a relationship. Instead of having a one-decade window where women choose motherhood, it now seems to span three decades. I have single friends in their mid-thirties thinking about freezing their eggs in case they don't meet that special someone before they're forty; another woman I know worked for two years with a surrogate mother to have a child. Lesbian women are entering the fertility clinics and adoption offices in record numbers. A student of mine in her forties recently starting going to acupuncture, doing yoga, and trying any other alternative techniques she could find after trying unsuccessfully to conceive for two years.

After we spoke, Ruggies called to let me know that she's taking a step to regain her sense of self during such a high-stress period of her life. Although it seemed like an indulgence, she signed up for a private yoga session with a well-known yoga teacher in Manhattan. Her goal? To learn some basic relaxation and breathing techniques to help her cope with the generalized anxiety she feels on a daily basis. Although it's a small step, I could tell she felt empowered by the decision and anticipated the upcoming date. As I tell my yoga students, one small step is all it takes. Like Ruggies, we can start with one breath and take it from there.

Faith's Story: The Sandwich Generation

One of the most stressful times in a woman's life can be taking care of elderly parents. I watched my mother take care of her parents for seven long years, and I witnessed the incredible amount of stress it caused and stamina it took. The "sandwich generation," which is composed of those who take care of their children and their older parents, has morphed as the traditional family has shifted. With people living longer, and multiple marriages on the rise, the number of women caretaking seems to be growing exponentially—one "sandwicher" I interviewed took care of her two children, both parents, *and* an elderly grandmother!

My mother talked to me about the trials of this period of her life, which started in her early forties. As my sister and I entered our teen years, her parents entered their golden age. My grandmother's health deteriorated and my grandfather Harry was diagnosed with Alzheimer's, which left my mother to wrestle with doctors, tend to emergencies, handle their Medicare, and even help them with their food shopping—while running a household and working full-time. When the stress from this became too intense, my grandparents moved from Brooklyn to our suburban New Jersey town. The proximity alleviated some stress created from constantly driving to Brooklyn and dealing with matters from afar, but it also meant that my mother became involved on a daily basis.

My mother's brother helped out; he lived about two hours away and supported my mother by visiting every weekend. They made decisions about medical care together. But, she recalls, "I was the daughter, and they needed to live near me. When things got really bad, I would fill him in and consult, but I was the main physical doer."

Tips for Dealing with High-Stress Situations

Find a sacred space.

Create rituals.

Call on your friends.

Find a support group.

Get professional help for depression.

Talk to someone who has been through it.

Look for the opportunity for growth.

Stay positive.

Connect with nature.

Exercise.

The stress came on several levels. First, the physical stress took its toll. My mother needed to manage the household, get us where we needed to go, and run around to various appointments, pharmacies, and meetings. The stress got increasingly worse as the years went on and her parents became more debilitated. My mom remembers getting a lot of viruses during that time, which forced her to slow down and stop.

The next level of stress stemmed from the emotional strain of watching her parents lose their autonomy. "I somehow always felt guilty that I still wasn't doing enough for them, but over the years they needed more and more." The guilt spilled over into how she felt about the rest of us; she worried that maybe she involved us too much, didn't spend enough time with us, neglected her relationship with my father.

Mentally, the stress came on strong when she had to make important decisions for her parents. "I didn't want to take over and overstep my boundaries," she says. "I respected my mother's judgment and I didn't want to usurp her authority. It does happen that you become more of the parental figure for your own parents, and that's a change, a change in your life. You lose your sense of self—you become this person who is just there for everyone else. It's stressful thinking you have to make medical decisions, have to use your judgment, and you are always second-guessing. Those medical decisions are stressful—it's always there; it never leaves your mind."

During those years, one thing came after another for my grandparents. A bad reaction to a pill. A broken shoulder. A car accident. Emergency medical situations. An unstable home nurse. Admission to a nursing home. Each one of these things threw my mother into a new realm of overdrive.

She turned to her inherent connection to the divine for help. "I was always trying to feel God's presence so that I would feel supported," recalls my mother of her caretaker period. "I didn't have an organized religion, but I felt what's meant to be is meant to be. I realized that I don't control things; I'm just here to help. The big picture is just what's happening. I always felt some kind of spiritual connection, but it's hard to sustain sometimes. I never asked, *Why?* I didn't go there. It just was what it was."

My mother also says sometimes a breath of fresh air, literally, was all she needed when things got too much for her to bear. On the weekends, she tried to get away to a quieter place, whether it was an ashram or a place in the country.

Yet, she says, could she do it over again, she would make a few changes. These changes include prioritizing what's really important. Saying no when her stress levels reach a breaking point. Not doing every single nitty-gritty detail. Getting more help, through using a food delivery service or getting a part-time nurse sooner. And taking the time to de-stress, "realizing that it's not your responsibility to make their lives perfect, what's happening is happening, it's not my job to make their lives happy."

My mother says it took her years to recover after her parents' deaths. "But I felt a sense of relief," she says. "Even though I missed them very much, I didn't feel that burden." Only then did she come back to herself. "I began to think, *What can I do with my time, what do I want to do? What about faith?* Getting back more to who I was without them was a very big change."

Uncovering Spirit

No matter in what stressful situation we find ourselves, many women yearn to find a sense of spiritual guidance underneath it all. I remember when I came to this realization. In college, a dear friend of mine committed suicide; I couldn't make sense of this tragic event and didn't understand how to proceed with my guilt and sadness. I realized I had to access something deeper and more profound than my surface level of reaction allowed me. I started to go to yoga class simply because I couldn't bear to be alone with my thoughts night after night. There, I learned to sit quietly and breathe. I found that the thing I dreaded most—facing my sadness and depression head on-was the thing that I most needed. By taking yoga and meditation classes, studying some of the ancient texts of yoga, and going to Buddhism classes with a friend, I learned that I am not my emotions, and that I could let them flow around me but not topple me over. I absorbed the idea that I had an indestructible force within me that, no matter what the circumstances, remained strong and solid. It was a revelation. Of course, the fear and anxiety didn't simply vanish, but these realizations helped me to gain clarity about my life and my decisions. These understandings also allowed me to feel more comfortable with myself as a young woman. And for the first time in my life, in yoga class I felt graceful rather than klutzy, which increased my confidence and allowed me to take chances I might not have taken.

Now I can see how transformative that period was for me. As with Jackie, Sarah, and my mother, it was a stressful situation— my friend's suicide—that allowed me to open up to exploring these other realms. Driven by desperation and depression, I learned to go a little deeper into my self with a little "s" and discover my Self. I'm grateful for that time in my life.

Connecting with spirit during high-stress times is a common thread that weaves through the narratives of many women's lives. My interviews revealed common themes among women. One of these is that nature seems to connect women of all ages and backgrounds to something sacred and profound. "Nature has always been a refuge for me," says Terry Ferretti, echoing the sentiments of many women I spoke with. Walking, golfing, even literally smelling the flowers provides an escape for us to lose ourselves, if only for a moment. "I get most connected to my sense of spirituality when I'm in nature—in the wind, birds, the natural world," says Keren Taylor. "Lately I've been trying to bring the natural world into my house, spend time with my dog, meditate, put plants in my house—trying to foster it instead of putting it off and saying, 'Oh, I'll do that in the summer.'"

Organized religion also helps us move from stress to spirit. These days, even those who've strayed from their childhood religion find that they can just extract the parts that work for them. Some go for the music, the community, the sermon. Others realize that all religions say fundamentally the same thing: Trust God. Love your neighbor. Go inward. Underneath it all, whether you call it religion or spirituality, it comes down to faith. During high-stress periods, connecting with a religion can actually mean better health. Recent studies have linked religious involvement to lower blood pressure, better immunity, lower rates of depression, higher survival rates following cardiac surgery, and greater longevity. One large study in *The American Journal of Public Health* followed more than five thousand Californians for twenty-eight years: Those who attended religious services at least once a week had a 23 percent lower risk of dying during the study period than those who attended less frequently, even after the researchers controlled for lifestyle factors and social support.[4]

A simple sense of gratitude can calm us down and help us transform our stress into spirit. Saying thank you for a beautiful day, a loving family, or a meal helps us put things into perspective. Terry Ferretti explains how she deals with living geographically far apart from her big Italian family: "Of course I miss them. But I have a wonderful husband who adores me, two great kids, and a fabulous grandson," she says. "Just thinking of my grandson, Keegan, makes me smile. When things are tough mentally or physically, I find a place to volunteer my time. I did the soup kitchen when both girls left home, and it made me stop and think about everything I have."

Even though it can be a major source of stress, work can also connect us with that sense of spirituality and wonder. For Keren, who works with adolescent girls, spirituality doesn't exist separately from the rest of her life. "You feel like there is some growth that takes place—you affect them and they affect you—that is powerful and part of my life on a daily basis. That doesn't just have to happen while you are sitting on a cushion." Feeling this kind of deep connection to work doesn't only happen to women who work in social services or nonprofits. Whether we are balancing a budget or drawing up plans for a new house, most of us want to feel as though we're doing something positive for ourselves and the world.

This gives us a sense of purpose and pride, a feeling that we are all part of the big picture, which helps to fuel our personal lives, self-confidence, and sense of meaning.

Of course, finding work that leaves you spiritually invigorated, rather than drained, is a delicate balance. On the one hand, work that involves helping others makes us feel that we are connected to humanity and that we are fulfilling our life's purpose. But the downside is that this kind of work can leave us feeling depleted. As women, we are often "givers." We feel much empathy for the suffering around us. And as women in overdrive, we tend to overdo it. I often look at my mother as an example. As a social worker for forty years, she helped innumerable people of all walks of life: children struggling in school, girls battling eating disorders, couples having difficulties in their relationships, women fighting breast cancer, families of people dealing with elderly, sick parents.

But the work, as noble as it is, took a toll on my mother. Many women in overdrive who have fulfilling careers also have a hard time leaving the office or leaving their work behind at the end of the day. I've seen friends doing amazing work, but they burn out because of how much they give. So in order to have this kind of meaningful work fuel our sense of connection, women tell me it's important to cultivate a healthy balance. A main theme I've heard is learning to say no. When already giving so much of themselves, women are often asked to work evenings and weekends and do other things that leave them feeling frazzled and unbalanced. Only through creating boundaries can our work help us feel connected with spirit, rather than disconnected from our bodies and our true nature.

Other ways women connect with our spirit side? Exercising, eating well, and learning to prioritize what is important to get done. Learning to say no and embracing our imperfections. Taking care of ourselves by meditating, taking baths, and creating a sacred space where we can retreat when we need to slow down and ask ourselves the big questions. Learning to laugh. Doing breathing exercises. Getting enough sleep. Looking at stress as an opportunity that can truly transform our whole experience as we put ourselves back together more wholly.

Life's Little Stresses

Volumes have been written about stress and its physical and emotional effects. Its impact on how we feel is profound. When you look at the causes of low energy, listlessness, and fatigue, stress is often the first culprit. Just dealing with everyday life can zap our resources. Stress can't always be avoided; life is unpredictable, and we need to be flexible when dealing with big changes like a move, divorce, or new job and even kinder and more compassionate to ourselves when dealing with the illness of a parent or the death of a friend or family member. But just the right amount of stress can actually be a good thing. If I didn't have deadlines for my work, I probably wouldn't get as much done as I do when I know an impending date looms. Stress motivates us and strengthens our determination to be accurate and responsible. But we often overlook the effects of life's *little* stresses, which accumulate and leave us drained and depleted without our really understanding the cause.

This morning, I got into my car to do some errands. I turned on the morning news, ran over a pothole, and glared at a fellow driver who barged across a four-way stop ahead of her turn. By the time I arrived at my first stop, the post office, I felt exhausted. The same actions could have resulted in a much different scenario: I turn on the classical music station instead of the news. I pay enough attention to the road that I avoid the pothole, and I forgive the woman for going through the stop—she could have been going to visit her husband in the emergency room after a heart attack. I just don't know.

When my head is clear enough, I try to remember the words of the Zen monk Thich Nhat Hanh about life on the road: "When we are driving, we tend to think of arriving and we sacrifice the journey for the sake of the arrival," he writes. "But life is to be found in the present moment, not the future." If we feel our stress levels soaring, Hahn suggests using visual cues such as a red stoplight as a reminder to come back to the moment. He says that although we might think of the red light as the enemy preventing us from achieving our goal, we can instead think of the light as a friend that helps us resist rushing and reminds us to return to a state of peacefulness. And even if you get cut off, cursed at, or confused about directions, he recommends acceptance as the final frontier. "It is useless to fight," says Hanh. "If you sit back and smile to yourself, you will enjoy the present moment and make everyone in the car happy."

Traffic is just one example of how we can actively work to reduce everyday stresses so that we feel relaxed at the end of the day instead of exhausted. We can use these techniques while at the DMV, in line at the grocery store, at the airport waiting for a flight. While walking from work to the car, engage in a walking meditation by counting your steps and staying aware of how your foot falls on the ground. When you wake up, you can take a moment or two to think about what you feel grateful for in your life, or imagine a white light of safety and healing around yourself or someone you love.

Another stressor for us women is excessive worrying. Again, a healthy amount is normal, but we can go overboard. As we age, it seems as if there's more to worry about: our health, our friends, the state of national affairs. But worrying generates a steady stream of low-grade anxiety, one that contributes to fatigue and lower quality of life than our potential. I find myself worrying about the strangest things: a mysterious illness that my husband might contract, a dearth of work a year from now. I've learned to label these things as "catastrophic thinking." Thinking of the worst-case scenario doesn't help anyone; it only hurts. As Mark Twain once famously said: "Some of the worst things in my life never happened."[5] I've found that labeling these worries, and then asking myself if they are legitimate concerns, helps to break the worrying cycle, that endless loop of worry that Daniel Goleman, author of *Emotional Intelligence*, calls "neural hijacking."[6]

We'd all love to be upbeat, high energy, and enthusiastic for much of our lives. Of course, this is a mere pipe dream. Reality dictates that we have external stresses and demands that we can't simply run from and responsibilities we need to fulfill. But it's many women's bane: We do too much. We pack our days with activities, can't say no to people, and convince ourselves that we must follow through on every bit on the to-do list. But this kind of determination has its consequences. As we age, we aren't as resilient as we used to be. Our bodies need time to regenerate, and many women say that although they manage to finish everything they started, the next day they feel depleted. Avoid this fate by understanding your body and how it works. Taking on a spiritual approach to stress will energize our bodies and minds. Beyond these handy tips, spiritual traditions suggest that we have infinite resources within us; we can handle whatever life puts in our way. Those who believe in God, a higher power, or a guiding force find that we get strength, direction, and love when we need it. One teacher told me that God doesn't give you anything that you can't handle. Knowing this gives us a powerful tool to not get so worked up about life's little stresses; we all know that we'll still have enough to deal with.

If a positive aspect of fatigue

exists, it's that our bodies are trying

to tell us something. Fatigue isn't just

an inevitable part of getting older;

it's a signal we need to heed.

If a positive aspect of fatigue exists, it's that our bodies are trying to tell us something. Fatigue isn't just an inevitable part of getting older; it's a signal that we need to heed. Although fatigue is a symptom of diseases like chronic fatigue, diabetes, heart disease, thyroid problems, and depression, most often it's simpler than that. Maybe we aren't getting enough exercise— or getting too much. Perhaps unresolved emotional issues are taking their toll. Too much sugar, stress, or work. Not pacing ourselves. Eating too much, or too little. Signs that tell us to change directions, shift gears, examine our circumstances. The highest approach, then, is to *thank* our fatigue for the opportunity to allow us to stop and reflect on the way we live our lives, make meaningful changes, and realign our bodies and minds.

As Maya Tiwari reminds us in her book *The Path of Practice:* "When you begin to live and move with the rhythms of nature, your mind becomes more lucid and more peaceful and your health improves. Your entire life becomes easier." And according to Tiwari, this extends even further out into the world: "Because women have always been the guardians of life's wholesome practices, when we strengthen our health and spiritual power, we also strengthen the health and wisdom of the men, children, and communities around us."[7]

chapter 4

capturing longevity

A captivating magazine article recently caught my eye. It was called "Finding the Fountain of Youth" and talked about biochemist and university professor Cynthia Kenyon, who is studying longevity in worms. Her lab research has increased the life span of tiny worms up to six times their normal life span by suppressing a certain "regulator" gene. Not only does this gene increase their longevity, but it also allows the worms to stay youthful for most of these extended years. It's a gene that could, she says, be able to do the same things in humans.[1]

"The public is absolutely fascinated by aging," says Kenyon.

And this is true. The public is obsessed with everything having to do with aging and achieving longevity. Beyond simply living a long time, like Kenyon's worms, we want our entire lives to be quality years filled with activity and growth. But what causes longevity? A decades-long study on aging by the John D. and Catherine T. MacArthur Foundation wanted to find out. This study, involving physicians, psychologists, gerontologists, sociologists, and other aging experts, set out to explain "why one eighty-two-year-old is on cross-country skis while another is in a wheelchair." The researchers wanted to figure out what causes these drastically different outcomes. Is it mostly our genetic disposition, as many people have asserted? Their conclusions have challenged the myth about aging: Their research found that only one-third of aging is determined by genes, while two-thirds depends on lifestyle and environment.[2] Basically, how we choose to live our lives is vastly more important than our heredity.

This is good news for women of all ages, from those of us in our thirties to women entering their twilight years. Rather than viewing aging as a process of losing control of our faculties, having our looks head south, and becoming increasingly dependent on others, this study is yet another reason to take control over how we live, accept responsibility for our lives, and ultimately become active participants in our own longevity.

When it comes to longevity, how we

choose to live our lives is vastly more

important than our heredity.

Obsession with Youth

My first real brush with feeling pressure to look young—and feeling the physical effects of aging—happened after I was hired to write an infomercial for a "miracle, anti-aging" face cream. I'd never done this kind of work before but thought I'd do a friend a favor. My job was to write a script for this "revolutionary" skin cream, a product that "reversed the signs of aging." For my research, the producer gave me tapes of women swearing by this product. I toiled for days over what to write without sounding cliché. How could I convince my fellow women that they needed to drop $80 on this cream?

Even more disturbing, however, was my own reaction over time. After reading the backup material over and over, I became convinced that my own skin was in rapid decline. I was suddenly sure that I had sunspots, sun damage, and dramatically oversized pores. Although I had never before thought about my skin that much, I started to seriously question my quick wash-and-rinse approach to skin care. I told myself I desperately needed a magic formula of Retin-A, a sophisticated sponge release system, and the highest grade of alpha hydroxys, all formulated by scientists and dermatologists after decades of testing. *I am almost thirty-four,* I told myself. I might wake up one day with crow's-feet and smile lines, looking haggard and twice my age. I tried to drop subtle hints to my producer so she would send me some of this miracle product to test out. After all, I reasoned, how could I write about something I hadn't tried? She didn't pick up on my hints, but still my doubt about my skin deepened. In a move embarrassing even to write about, I then decided to shell out the money and order the miracle cream—only to find that it wasn't on the market yet. Once I found out that my product was unattainable, the mania faded. My face looked fine. I continued to wash with the relatively inexpensive products I get at the health-food store, and I never really gave it another thought.

But this shift from believer to skeptic wasn't so good for my infomercial-writing career. After sending in my final script, I got a perfectly polite note from my producer to this effect: "Thanks for your copy. It's not exactly what we are looking for. I think it's better if we continue with another writer, but we'll let you know our needs in the future."

I've been fired from only one job—and this was it. Why couldn't I write a silly infomercial that convinced women that they desperately needed help looking younger? Getting fired is no fun, but I soon began to look at the fact as a source of pride. I wouldn't be a part of the machine that churns out messages about staying youthful, about how aging is bad and you must do everything in your power to stop it, or at least quell the tide.

My intention is to age with pride. That's easy for me to say, of course, because I'm still in my thirties. And since this work experience, I've noticed my own judgments about other women I come across with wrinkles or uneven skin. It's amazing to watch my mind. Although I feel so strongly about aging with pride, after decades of being bombarded with messages about staying young forever, they have seeped in unwittingly. Of all people, I should know. As a magazine editor, I've seen what goes on behind the scenes. With the standard use of Photoshop on magazine covers and spreads, our view of "normal" has become totally skewed. With this technology, you can skim inches off a model's waist and thighs. You can erase blemishes of any kind. You can add cleavage. It's frightening.

It seems like a tide that's impossible to stem and one that leads the average woman to feel mighty self-conscious about the natural flow of aging. We all know absolutely ravishing women who have low self-esteem. We undercut each other and compare our physical attributes—number of gray hairs, weight loss and gain, bags under the eyes. We don't seize the opportunity to band together and say we aren't going to take this anymore. Imagine a world where women support one another and reject these notions of aging.

I'm not saying you shouldn't take care of your skin; however, the emphasis on appearances should stem from a desire for self-care, rather than competition with our beautifully Botoxed

Risk Factors for Melanoma[3]

1. You've spent a lot of time in the sun and/or had multiple blistering burns as a child.
2. You have fair skin, blue eyes, red or blond hair.
3. You have a lot of moles on your body.
4. You know of two or more family members with melanoma.

neighbor. Excessive early exposure to the sun leads to photoaging, which results in premature wrinkles, spots, dry skin, discoloration, and freckles. Beyond being a purely cosmetic issue, half the new cancers in the United States are skin cancers, affecting a million people each year. Melanoma is the seventh most common cancer in women and causes more than three-quarters of skin cancer deaths.

As a woman in overdrive, I look back to when my overdrive started. I now realize that I always strove to be the best and go a little overboard, even at a young age. I remember how important it was to come back from vacations as a teenager looking tan. I wanted to look better and healthier than anyone else, and I thought a deep, dark tan was the way to do it. Although it makes me cringe to think about it now, I spent many vacations slathering on baby oil and sitting in the hot sun for hours. And now I have the sunspots and freckles to show for it. Ironically, the very thing that drove me to look the "best" has turned on me! Recently, I went to get a facial. My aesthetician clucked and shook her head after examining my face under the magnified mirror as I listened in embarrassment. "You need a regimen! You *must* have a regimen!" she repeated. I noticed the two sides of myself debate. One side was skeptical; after all, she wanted me to buy her products. But the other was noticeably fearful. Maybe I did need a regimen. Maybe it was too late for me and my spotty skin.

Factors in Photoaging

1. Degree of sun exposure
2. Skin pigment
3. Skin type
4. Cigarette smoking
(Photoaging doesn't have to happen as you age.)[4]

These days, hopefully, we are educated enough about the dangers of ultraviolet rays on our skin to avoid going out in the sun with a thick layer of oil. But women in overdrive really need to stay conscious of photoaging and skin cancer. It's not too late for me, but many other women don't think about the negative effects of the sun before it's too late. Despite the mounting evidence, why do we choose to ignore it? Women in overdrive tend to live life to the fullest. We're out there jogging, playing tennis, walking. We go on vacations to sunny locales and spend weekends outdoors. In the moment, it's easy to forget about wearing that hat or putting on sunscreen. It's important to remember that we can live life exuberantly in the present and still keep the future in mind while we do it.

Make Your Skin Glow[5]

1. Don't smoke. The chemicals from smoke and the constant pursing of your lips add to aging skin.
2. If you diet, take off weight slowly so you don't get saggy and stretchy skin, which happens as your skin loses elasticity as you age.
3. Get enough sleep. Sleep mends your skin.

The Age Chronicles

I was able to remove myself from the constant messages out there that were telling me that I wasn't okay. I had broken the chain of comparing myself to a twenty-five-year-old. I had looked around and used my sense, rather than the societal messages of beauty I see all around me. At thirty-five, this was relatively easy to do. But what about when I turn forty, fifty, and sixty? The confluence of two things—an increasingly consumer-driven society and my own personal aging process—just might put me over the edge. Even now, I see reality shows that turn ugly ducklings into swans, a plastic surgery epidemic, and women obsessed with weight and exercise. I see how cultural pressures to stay young create needless unhappiness and suffering and make us feel interminably incomplete. From talking to many women, I know the messaging becomes only more intense as we age. At my age, I see how we are pressed to achieve a certain narrow view of beauty. But as we age, I also see that images of older women barely exist in the popular culture. They have been swept under the table, invisible and invalidated.

Forties: Pressure's On

I asked Sarah Nesson for some insight about her experience of aging. After all, forty-one is just around the corner for me. Sarah is a statuesque, attractive woman with gray streaks in her dark hair; she's obviously toned and healthy from her regular practices of swimming and practicing yoga.

"I'm more aware of the aging process than I ever have been, which makes sense because I'm in the middle of my life," she says. "It's probably the combination of losing a parent and turning forty. I'm also aware of changes in my appearance: I'm getting gray hair and lines in my face that I know aren't going to go away. I also have noticed a difference in my level of energy, and I'm realizing that I'm probably not going to have a family; now I don't think that would be possible."

I asked Sarah if she felt pressure, in her forties, to look young. "I don't dye my hair," she says. "No one my age has even one gray hair. Everybody dyes it. I'm just aware that I no longer fit, I no longer look as youthful as I used to, and I'm not in that pool of women considered to be young and attractive anymore. It's not really pressure, but I'm aware that I'm transitioning out of what is considered our more beautiful age. That makes me sad, because whenever I look at other women my age and older, I think they look very beautiful with lines on their faces. It's easy to think this of others, but it's harder to transfer to myself—even when I'm not smiling, there are still lines there! Hopefully one day we'll be like in some cultures where the more lines you have, the more beautiful you are considered."

Fifties: The Invisible Woman

Moving on from this transitional phase of the forties, women in their fifties tell me that they feel "invisible" and "less than." Fifty-two-year-old Marsha Hultberg had this to stay about the cultural attitudes about longevity and aging: "All of a sudden you feel invisible on the street; it's the stereotypical thing you hear. I am a very attractive woman and used to turn a lot of heads. I'm still attractive, but I'm older now. I look at my body and I don't recognize it anymore. All of a sudden, everything changes: Your vision goes, your bones start hurting, the aches and the pains in the morning, your teeth turn yellow. It's like, wow! In my head I am still twenty-five or thirty."

Hultberg says she isn't fighting aging, but she isn't exactly embracing it either. "I was a dancer for many years, and I had a fantastic body. I don't have it anymore. Everything has gone south. My upper arms are flabby, like my mother's. It's creepy! When did that happen? Overnight? I recently worked with a personal trainer, and when I told him my age, he couldn't believe it. He told me I should be proud of my body."

Unfortunately, many women feel shame rather than pride. It seems as if the women I meet are still on diets or obsessed with youth. Hultberg continued: "Well, I *should* be proud of my body; I have a good mind, I should have a good self-image, but because of our society, I am not proud of my body. I'm not perfect. We are so conditioned to think we need to be perfect. I had my teeth whitened because I was going out to meet someone. But we need to celebrate who we are."

Sixties: A Pivotal Point

At sixty-four, my mother represents women in their sixties for whom achieving longevity and aging gracefully have been lifelong priorities. I remember when she interviewed for a job at age sixty-one. I reviewed her résumé for her, and I noticed she had omitted a few of her very early jobs. When I asked her about this, she told me that she didn't want the dates to go so far back so that people could decipher her age. I was surprised; my mother had never expressed any reticence about revealing her age before. But she told me that it wasn't her vanity; she just thought that people have a lot of internal discrimination when it comes to hiring people in their sixties. "First, they think you won't stay long because you are going to retire soon," she says. "But mainly, when people hear you are in your sixties, they have an automatic mindset. They pigeonhole you and put you in a certain group." Ironically, because my mother looks so young, she is experiencing a kind of delayed reaction: Others now put her in the "fifties" group. "In general people know that I'm older, but they don't know I'm in my sixties."

As a younger person, I had never thought of this. But it made sense: Although it's technically illegal, many people would rather hire someone they perceive as "young and energetic" than someone "older and slower."

At first, my mother was reluctant to admit to any pressure she felt to look young. She kept saying things like, "It's hard to say if I feel pressure" or, "Pressure? I wouldn't call it *pressure*." She had a hard time differentiating between the pressure she put on herself and the pressure from society. I argued that it's the same thing: If we didn't feel cultural pressure, why would we pressure ourselves to look different than we do? She called me a day later to admit to more pressure than she let on. "It's such a part of me," she said, "I don't even realize that I feel it every day."

As for her thoughts on longevity, my mother says she wouldn't consider plastic surgery because of her commitment to health. In other words, surgery and Botox, whose long-term effects are both unknown, just don't seem like healthy options to her. "I would just learn to live with it," she says of any visible signs of aging that might happen in the future.

Despite outside pressures, she said that there reaches a point when you know that no matter what you do, you realize can't get back to how you once looked. "I stay fit and slim, but I'm not crazy with it," she says. "I don't do anything for my thighs or arms, for instance. I say, look, I'm allowed. I'm sixty-four; I don't have to tone my arms, I am not going to appear nude, if I wear short sleeves that's fine. There is a part of me that's accepted my body, that this is a part of normal life and that's okay."

She reached this turning point in her fifties, when she realized that self-acceptance was more important than trying to fit a younger mold. "I'm not going to go out of my way to appear in a bathing suit. People look at you, they know you are older.

But within myself I'm comfortable." Many women I spoke with seemed to mirror my mother's conflicted feelings about longevity. Is she comfortable, or not? Does she care what people think, or not? Does she feel real outside pressure? These conflicts exist within most women during their entire lives, and it seems that the aging process heightens these inner tensions. "Living in the city, I sometimes get jealous of the young people I see. I was once there once, and now I'm not. It's fun to be young."

Lessons from Centenarians

Monika White, president of the Center for Healthy Aging in Santa Monica, California, found some key similarities among people who have lived to be 100.

CENTENARIANS:

1. are not obese
2. rarely smoke
3. have low incidence of age-related health problems like stroke, heart attacks, cancer, diabetes
4. handle stress better than average
5. have a sense of humor
6. feel a sense of hope about the future
7. stay engaged with interests and hobbies
8. have the ability to cope with loss and go on with life

The Plastic Surgery Epidemic

Oprah loves makeovers. I've discovered this over the years. At the four o'clock hour, when many people need a lift from the workday, instead of having chocolate or a mocha latte, I sneak away for my favorite indulgence, *The Oprah Winfrey Show*. I've been shocked to notice how many shows feature people who've had plastic surgery. The story always goes something like this: A woman in her fifties, maybe recently divorced and frumpy as can be, decides to turn her life around. A few tens of thousands of dollars later, after liposuction and LASIK surgery and a boob job and face-lift and teeth whitening, Oprah gives her guest a designer wardrobe and she struts onstage. The change in appearance is often dramatic; the woman usually gets a standing ovation. Then she tells the audience how much better she feels. She's had her first date in twenty years, has more energy, gets seductive looks from men on the street, and has decided to take up new hobbies and travel around the world.

What surprises me most is the degree to which Oprah supports plastic surgery. By featuring such women, she ultimately spreads the plastic surgery gospel. And the applause and accolades only serve to reinforce the idea that radical surgery validates a woman's existence. I really love what Oprah does otherwise; over the years she has stood for empowering women, taking charge of your life, and finding a sense of spirit and meaning in your life. So why the contradiction? Ultimately, I think Oprah's conflict is my conflict: If a woman feels better about herself, then what's wrong with a little nip and tuck? Who am I to say that feeling better about yourself is bad? But

it's deeper than that. Having major, and often dangerous, surgery doesn't seem to be the answer. But it feels so big and
daunting to change the tide in plastic surgery; it would mean
taking on the entire cultural ideals of beauty. It would mean
telling ourselves that we look good enough in our natural state,
that we can have new hobbies and successes and sexy looks
without having to radically alter our appearance.

The tension is real: Fight it or join it? Like Oprah and I,
Marsha Hultberg feels this pull. "If I had any extra money I
would do a little lift and take ten years off," she says. "It's vanity. I would never have thought I would do it, but now that
I'm here—fifty-two years old—I would. But it's not my belief
system; that's not who I am."

Think It Over: What If?

According to the American Society of Plastic Surgeons (ASPS),
10.2 million cosmetic plastic surgery procedures were performed in the United States in 2005, up 11 percent from the
previous year.[6] In addition, more than 5.4 million reconstructive
plastic surgery procedures were performed last year. According to the ASPS, the top five surgical procedures were liposuction, nose reshaping, breast augmentation, eyelid surgery, and
tummy tuck. That's a lot of elective surgeries. Indeed, plastic
surgery makes some women feel better about themselves. But
what factors should be taken into consideration when thinking
about plastic surgery?

Reasons for Doing It

Before delving into plastic surgery, it's important to take some time to think about your motivations. Are you doing this for yourself, or is your partner pressuring you?

Are you in denial that you are aging?

For many women, soul-searching results in the decision not to go through with it. For others, taking time out to think only strengthens their resolve. But the most important thing is not to make a hasty decision. Plastic surgery is just that—surgery. It comes with very real risks of infection, excess bleeding, and long recovery times. Psychologically, surgery can be devastating if your expectations aren't met. After spending so much time and energy on the surgery, not to mention money, some women come to realize what they want to "fix" or "perfect" is more of an internal issue than an external one. Unrealistic expectations about your new, "perfect" self can lead to a major letdown when you discover that you are still the same old you.

Price

What is youth worth to you? Many women skimp and save to afford a new look. A full face-lift costs $15,000–$20,000 and requires a few weeks off.[7] Even if the financial aspect isn't important, think about the price in terms of your time and level of comfort. It might take months for the swelling to subside, and some women complain of fatigue for up to two months after surgery.

Outcome

We've all seen the actresses on television who look distorted and fake. In their sixties, they don't have a wrinkle in sight and their faces look unnaturally smooth and shiny. If you consider plastic surgery, make sure you don't overdo it!

Menopause and Longevity

It makes sense that longevity is on the minds of women going through menopause. After all, menopause is a very physical sign that life is progressing. The biggest thing I've learned as a younger woman about menopause is how wildly different it is for everyone. At my stage, this sounds strikingly similar to another major physical change for women—pregnancy. Every woman I've spoken with who's gone through pregnancy has had a wildly different experience. Some had morning sickness for six months; others had none. Some felt energetic and glowing most of the time; others felt fatigued and crabby. The list goes on, and the same goes for menopause: Some women have virtually no symptoms and fly through it. Others find menopause to be a gradual process, starting with perimeno pause that lasts for years and gradually segueing into full-blown menopause.

"Emotionally, it was rough," says Marsha Hultberg. "My mother was gone and I couldn't talk to her about it. She was one of these women who didn't notice it; she was in denial and very depressed, and my sister and I both had extreme reactions to it." Extreme reactions aren't uncommon. "Becoming middle-aged is overwhelming," adds Hultberg. "It's a marker of becoming old and feeling past tense, not vital, less attractive—all of those things. Of course, these things aren't true, but they're the things that loom in the back of your mind."

For my own mother, menopause was a gradual process—and a marker of when she really started to think about her aging process. "Menopause was a difficult time for me," she says. "I put on a few pounds and I looked drawn. I had different physical things happen. I guess it's like the start of aging, but I think I aged slowly. Even my body didn't start to sag until a few years ago. My hair didn't turn gray. I'd say the mid to late fifties was a lot of change, but the big change was going into my sixties. That's a big number."

Psychologically, menopause throws some into turmoil, the proverbial "midlife crisis" that happens when we can no longer have children, particularly for women who strongly identify themselves as fertile caretakers of the earth.

For others, menopause and midlife are signs of a new beginning. Such is the case for fifty-year-old Patricia Karnowski, an acupuncturist and clinical psychiatrist whose hysterectomy threw her into menopause last year. Ever since a friend had a vision that Patricia would live until she was eighty-eight, she's felt that even though she's in the middle of her life, she still has a long way to go. "I have some time, but I can also feel the end," she says. "I want to be as healthy as I can be for as long as I can, and I never thought about it like that before. I realize that I have some influence on my own longevity, and I am planning for this next half of life in a way that I never ever thought to in a real

Live Long and Prosper

Healthy aging doesn't have to come under a surgeon's knife. Lifestyle changes and adjustments are key to living longer and healthier. Among the positive steps you can take are these:

1. Get involved in your community.
2. Create social networks.
3. Maintain a positive attitude.
4. Eat right.
5. Exercise.
6. Get enough sleep.
7. Keep your mind active and engaged.

way. Now it feels real. I like the feeling that I'm in the world and can have an influence."

She plans to "do her part" in the world by traveling to India and Africa next year to help out with disadvantaged populations. "I don't know if it's because of my age or my hysterectomy, but I can feel there is an end to life," she says. In fact, she rails against the term "midlife crisis," which she says sounds too negative. Instead, she prefers to call it simply a "shift" or a "big change."

Could Karnowski's attitude about aging be the *real* fountain of youth? Celebrating who we are, at any age, allows us
to think young and feel motivated to do what it takes to stay
that way. The MacArthur Study makes it clear: Our lifestyle is
just as important as our genes. If you believe in the powerful
mind/body connection, which says that our thoughts have the
power to influence our body and our wellness, then we can
become cocreators in our own longevity. As my husband says in
his usual succinct matter: "What we focus on expands." What
I've learned from women older than I is that focusing on feeling happy and peaceful and accepting creates just that kind of
life—no matter what your circumstances.

"I have a real sense of gaining as I age," says Sarah Nesson,
"because I feel more mature and settled and at peace in my life,
and at peace with myself. There is a sense of knowing who I am,
a sense of how to nourish myself and contribute in the world.
That has deepened, along with a sense of weaving together a
lot of the strands of my life, my music, community building,
weaving them together and offering them."

Celebrating who we are, at any age,

allows us to think young and feel motivated

to do what it takes to stay that way.

chapter 5

understanding complementary and alternative medicine

The other day, I went to a nearby pharmacy to drop off a prescription for a friend. While I waited, I drank a cup of tea and did some research on pregnancy at a computer kiosk. I browsed among the yoga equipment, natural cosmetics, organic fruit, and dietary supplements. As I walked down the aisles, I looked at fact sheets that listed the pros and cons of certain products like vitamin C. I looked at the upcoming list of in-store practitioners: ayurvedic doctors, herbalists, and massage therapists, a discussion on a newly published book on Tibetan Buddhism, and demonstrations like "Mind/Body: Introduction to the Rosen Method." If I'd had the inclination, I could've gotten a chair massage and taken a class on tai chi chuan.

Although unusual, a pharmacy that combines complementary and Western medicine makes perfect sense. Driving the demand for this new model of pharmacy are the Baby Boomers, who came of age during the open-minded 1960s and must now struggle with the "less is more" policies of HMOs, which provide little if any preventive care. So it's no surprise that this generation has turned to complementary treatments. According to the AARP Public Policy Institute, eighty-three million Americans have used some form of complementary and alternative medicine (CAM), and the largest segment of CAM users is the fifty-to-sixty-four age group.[1]

It makes sense that these consumers, highly educated and proactive about their health, are spurring on a new model of care that blends East and West. "Boomers are approaching health in a new way from the previous generation," says AARP spokesman Mark Beach. "They are willing to look at alternative medicines and explore other healthcare options."

But it's not only Baby Boomers interested in combining the best of both worlds. A 2004 government survey shows that 36 percent of U.S. adults age eighteen and over use some form of CAM, which includes herbal medicine, acupuncture, chiropractic, vitamin therapy, and energy work.[2]

"The lines between mainstream and counterculture are pretty blurred," says Russell Precious, vice president of design and branding at Pharmaca, another "integrative pharmacy." Pharmaca's stores are staffed with naturopathic doctors, nurses, nutritionists, herbalists, homeopaths, and aestheticians. Pharmacists are highly knowledgeable about supplement use and drug/herb interactions. To maintain a neighborhood feel, the pharmacies include spaces for people to relax, sit, drink tea, or study.

Indeed, the groundswell of interest in holistic health and wellness has gained momentum over the past ten years. Across the country, complementary centers attached to major hospitals offer visualization, massage, yoga, and breathwork. Stores like Whole Foods have become tremendously popular and profitable, and even the most mainstream among us can be found at the acupuncturist's office for treatment of one ailment or another.

According to the AARP Public Policy

Institute, 8.3 million Americans have

used some form of complementary

and alternative medicine (CAM),

and the largest segment of CAM

users is the 50 to 64 age group.

As these two worlds meld together, however, things have the potential to get a little confusing. In my pregnancy, I have often felt barraged by the number of choices available to me. Many examples exist, but I'll use the ultrasound as mine. In my mother's day, nobody got an ultrasound. Now it seems that an ultrasound is standard procedure for expectant families. But just because the technology exists doesn't mean we need to use it. So I had to educate myself on the pros and con

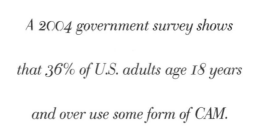

A 2004 government survey shows

that 36% of U.S. adults age 18 years

and over use some form of CAM.

of ultrasound: Is it safe? Would I terminate the pregnancy if I found a problem? Do I really want to know if there is a problem that can't be remediated? These are individual choices and ones that generations of women before me weren't faced with. In addition to these kinds of decisions, I also want to do my best to prepare my body for the rigors of labor. I started going to see an acupuncturist to balance my energy and have less fatigue. Then my lower back started to hurt. I found out about a great chiropractor who works with pregnant women, so I started going to her. My midwife suggested I get a few prenatal massages for relaxation. And my regular yoga classes help to strengthen and stretch my body. Of course, I couldn't keep up with all of these different treatments while at the same time going to my regular practitioner for prenatal care. Finally, I remembered that there isn't one path to health. In the interest of time and money, I would have to choose a route and stick to it.

And this is true for all conditions and ailments, at any stage of life, with any condition. It's easy to feel overwhelmed with the daily barrage of products at the pharmacy, the never-ending stream of studies released that often contradict one another, and advice from our well-meaning friends. But sometimes information overload can lead to paralysis. In fact, many of us can get almost obsessive in our quest for information because we live in a society of overwhelming choice. I always think about going to a little pharmacy in Greece the day after my husband had some digestive problems. The pharmacist walked out to greet us and we told her the problem. She disappeared behind a door. A moment later, she reemerged with the solution in the form of what looked like a tiny pill consisting of concentrated prune juice extract. There were no rows and rows of products in colorful packages, all claiming to be the most effective. The simplicity surprised me. One treatment for one ailment.

But back in the States, we are confronted with the overwhelming number of options—even more so now that we have both complementary and Western medicine accessible to us. Instead of buying everything on the shelf, we have to make a decision. So how do we do this in the midst of all of the choices? If we aren't careful, we can get caught up in the same spinning wheel of feeling overwhelmed that we see in other areas of our lives, which only hinders our health rather than helps it. So as we take advantage of the plethora of choices available to us, it's important to avoid the pattern by educating ourselves about the options, and then quieting down to listen as we ask ourselves the question: *What is the best solution for me and my unique situation?*

The problem arises, however, when we run in overdrive and don't take the time to slow down and consider what's best for us. When constantly in this state, we seem to feel that the more

we do, see, and buy, the more successful and accomplished we
have become! Objectively we know this is absurd. But we are
so caught up in this mindset that it's hard to step out of it.

Tracy W. Gaudet, MD, author of the book *Consciously
Female: How to Listen to Your Body and Your Soul for a Lifetime
of Healthier Living*, puts it this way: "Knowledge itself is a
powerful thing. You can—and should—learn as much as you
want about a particular health practice or treatment decision. It's also useful to gather perspectives from different
people, for example those who have been through a particular experience before. It's valid to seek second opinions and
to learn about the full range of options for treating a given
problem." But Gaudet points out that this isn't enough. "All
of the external information in the world cannot tell you
about *your* experience," she says. "Only you can know that. If
we acknowledge and increase our awareness around the ways
that we are in flux every day—if we begin to pay attention
and tune in to the ways our bodies, our emotions, and our
intellects shift throughout our cycles as well as throughout
the phases of our lives—the result will be a prosperous marriage of information and consciousness. We can, very simply, make better choices about our lives. And that makes our
existence better and easier."[3]

Do you want to take a prescription medication or homeopathic tablets? Take an over-the-counter drug or apply a hot
water bag to your chest? Sweat it out on a long hike or spend all
day on the couch? These are questions only you can answer by
tuning in to your body to see what feels right as you consider
what kind of therapy you feel most comfortable with.

It's easy to feel overwhelmed with

the daily barrage of products at the

pharmacy, the never-ending stream of

studies released that often contradict

one another, and advice from well-

meaning friends. Sometimes information

overload can lead to paralysis.

National Center for Complementary and Alternative Medicine breaks down CAM techniques into five categories:[4]

1. ALTERNATIVE MEDICAL SYSTEMS

These are built upon complete systems of theory and practice, often ones that have evolved apart from and earlier than the conventional medical approach used in the United States:

➔ Homeopathic medicine

➔ Naturopathic medicine

➔ Traditional Chinese medicine

➔ Ayurveda

2. MIND/BODY INTERVENTIONS

These techniques are designed to enhance the mind's capacity to affect the body:

➔ Meditation

➔ Prayer

➔ Therapies that use creative outlets, such as art, music, and dance

3. BIOLOGICALLY BASED THERAPIES

These use substances found in nature, such as herbs, foods, and vitamins:

→ Dietary supplements

→ Herbal products

4. MANIPULATIVE AND BODY-BASED METHODS

These are based on manipulation and/or movement of one or more parts of the body:

→ Chiropractic

→ Osteopathic

→ Massage

5. ENERGY THERAPIES

These involve the use of energy fields:

→ Qigong

→ Reiki

→ Therapeutic touch

→ Bioelectromagnetic-based therapies involving the unconventional use of electromagnetic fields, such as pulsed fields, magnetic fields, and alternating-current or direct-current fields

What Is Complementary and Alternative Medicine?

With the addition of CAM to our menu of medical and treatment options, it's important to understand exactly what this is. According to the National Center for Complementary and Alternative Medicine (NCCAM), complementary and alternative medicine is "a group of diverse medical and health care systems, practices, and products that are not presently considered to be part of conventional medicine."[5] Complementary and alternative medicine do not shun traditional medicine. On the contrary, alternative medical approaches open up the spectrum to a wider range of options. Someone diagnosed with cancer, for example, can choose either a specialized diet or radiation and chemotherapy. A major point of alternative medicine is that one size does not fit all; instead of prescribing one pill for one ailment, alternative medicine seeks to work with the patient's unique needs and come up with the plan that works the best for him or her.

More and more people are using CAM as the first line of defense against common ailments, from colds to canker sores. This has become much easier with the widespread availability of information and the boom in "mainstream" health-food stores. As we become more knowledgeable, we also feel more confident in our choices. A few months ago, I had a problem with a tendon in my hand. I went to a hand doctor, who showed me some gory pictures and told me I needed a cortisol shot and then surgery. I left his office feeling shocked. My hand hurt, but it didn't seem that drastic. So I made an appointment with my acupuncturist. After a few sessions, alternating ice and heat and using a homeopathic cream for inflammation, my symptoms have disappeared. Looking back on the experience, I am grateful that I was empowered to do this. Otherwise, I would've been on the operating table and probably taking antibiotics and other medicines that might have led to an imbalance in my body. Based on my experience, I also realize how many unnecessary surgeries are performed annually. It's good to use CAM as a first defense. In my situation, if CAM hadn't worked and I had continued to have serious pain, I might have opted for surgery down the line. But something simple worked, and I was able to prevent a lot of extra pain, expense, and recovery time.

More and more people are using CAM as the first line of defense against common ailments, from colds to canker sores.

You Decide: Conditions and Options for Healing

Over the decades, a woman's body inevitably goes through a multitude of changes and challenges. So what are the options for both more alternative approaches and the more mainstream modes of healing? To get you started, here are a few of the conditions many of us will go through over a lifetime, along with suggestions for both alternative and mainstream approaches for dealing with them. I want to stress that this is by no means an exhaustive list of treatments, but simply an outline to get you started on doing your own research. Each one of these conditions could fill a book in itself. The purpose here is just to get you on your way. Please know that many of the herbs and supplements I mention have not been scientifically proven to work, and some of them can actually be harmful if taken in large quantities or if they interact with other drugs or medications you are taking. Many of the drugs and treatments also have serious side effects. Because this is just a preliminary list, I have not mentioned dosage, side effects, or interactions. That is something to work out with your own practitioner. Ultimately we must take our health into our own hands, weighing the risks and benefits and remembering that the choice is ours.

What's the Difference?

(NCCAM is sure to differentiate between the names.)[6]

→ Complementary medicine is used together with conventional medicine. An example of a complementary therapy is aromatherapy after surgery to help a patient heal and ease his or her pain.

→ Alternative medicine is used in place of conventional medicine. An example of an alternative therapy is a special diet to treat cancer instead of surgery, radiation, or chemotherapy.

→ Integrative medicine combines mainstream medical therapies and CAM therapies that have been shown to be safe and effective.

Premenstrual Syndrome (PMS)

Maybe you just feel a bit out of sorts. Or perhaps you have debilitating cramps that keep you in bed. Just a few short decades ago, women who complained of symptoms before their period were given tranquilizers, antidepressants, or a hysterectomy.[7] Today, it's widely acknowledged that 60 to 85 percent of women experience some degree of PMS over their lifetime, while 5 percent of us are diagnosed with premenstrual dysphoric disorder (PMDD), a severe form that leaves us feeling emotionally or physically impaired.[8] Indeed, PMS is no longer a shameful or hidden condition, and at some time in our lives, most of us have suffered its symptoms—headaches, depression, moodiness, cravings, insomnia, difficulty concentrating, sore breasts, fluid retention, backaches, cramps, acne, irritability, constipation, or joint point. I could go on, since a whopping 150 PMS symptoms have been documented. Although every woman has her own unique experience, broadly defined, PMS is the combination of emotional and physical symptoms that begin a week or two before menstruation, continue until a period arrives, and recur in two out of every three menstrual cycles.

Although there are many theories, the most common cause of PMS involves a hormonal imbalance of estrogen and progesterone. Interestingly, the condition is more likely to occur in our thirties and early forties.[9] Researchers have various ideas about why, including the fact that women in this age range have more external factors contributing to hormonal shifts—pregnancy, miscarriage, a discontinuation of the birth control pill. Another reason cited is stress: Women in their thirties and forties often experience increased amounts of stress, including motherhood, care of elderly family members, and increased expectations at work.

PMS: Alternative Therapies

Herbs and teas

Chasteberry: Stimulates the production of progesterone.

Dandelion leaf: Reduces water retention.

Kava kava: Reduces irritability and anxiety.

Ginger-and-chamomile tea: Relieves headaches and menstrual cramps.

Passionflower tea: Relieves insomnia.

Cramp bark / Raspberry: Eases cramps.

Calcium

Studies show that a daily calcium supplement can help to reduce PMS symptoms such as irritability and anxiety, possibly because of its effect on mood-enhancing brain chemicals called neurotransmitters.

Vitamin B

Vitamin B, particularly B6, improves myriad symptoms of PMS.

Vitamins A and E

Help decrease pain and ease hormonal changes.

Magnesium

May help alleviate emotional symptoms, insomnia, fluid retention, and breast tenderness.

Reflexology

Applying manual pressure to specific points on the ears, hands, and feet may relieve some PMS symptoms.

Acupuncture

Many of the symptoms of PMS, including headaches, breast tenderness, and pain, are signs that the liver meridian is stagnant, according to Traditional Chinese Medicine (TCM). This "liver qi (life force) stagnation" means that your energy is not flowing properly. With acupuncture, you can address specific symptoms through points on the arms, legs, and abdomen. Alongside treatments, two herbs are helpful in getting the qi moving: don quai and xiao yao wan.

Exercise

We know it feels great to get moving when we feel emotionally or physically challenged. Indeed, research shows that regular exercise can reduce PMS symptoms. Exercise boosts endorphins, which in turn help relieve cramps and improve mood. Try walking, riding a bike, dancing at home, or practicing yoga or tai chi.

Natural progesterone

Commonly in the form of a cream or a pill, natural progesterone can help alleviate PMS symptoms if you are found to have low progesterone levels.

PMS: Mainstream Therapy

The birth control pill helps to ease PMS because it stabilizes the fluctuations of hormones. Women trying to get pregnant who don't want to go on the pill can try an estrogen patch, which delivers a continuous low dose of estradiol, supplementing your body's estrogen and stabilizing the estrogen/progesterone balance at the root of PMS. Another mainstream approach to PMS is an antidepressant like Serafem or Celexa.

Nutrition

Eating right and knowing what to avoid are key to managing PMS symptoms:

→ Avoid salt, which can lead to water retention.

→ Eat six small meals a day to avoid anxiety, irritability, and fatigue.

→ Balance your carbohydrate intake with a small amount of protein, vegetables, and/or fruit.

→ Keep food stashed close by to avoid dips in blood sugar.

→ Avoid caffeine, a stimulant that intensifies breast soreness and anxiety and interferes with sleep.

→ Avoid refined sugar, which may increase water retention and bloating.

→ Avoid alcohol, which can act as a depressant.

→ Drink lots of water; it alleviates bloating and helps avoid fatigue.

→ Eat complex carbohydrates like whole grain breads, pastas and cereals, sweet potatoes, brown rice, and fresh fruits and vegetables.

→ Add calcium to your diet, which may help with irritability. Try milk products like yogurt, ice cream, and cheese. Dark greens also help. Try broccoli, raw green or red cabbage, and cooked collards. Other good foods include salmon and sardines; soy products, such as tofu and soy milk; and calcium-fortified orange and grapefruit juices.

Fibromyalgia

Many of us have bad days where we feel achy and tired. But for others, this feeling goes beyond the normal scope of everyday wear and tear. Fibromyalgia is a chronic condition characterized by aching pain, stiffness, and tenderness in the muscles, tendons, and ligaments. It affects nearly 3.7 million Americans, or 5 percent of the population, mostly occurring in women of childbearing age. Despite the recent rise in its acceptance as a legitimate ailment, researchers don't know what causes fibromyalgia (beyond a few guesses, like a neurotransmitter imbalance or overly sensitive cells), and it seems to be currently one of the most mysterious and misunderstood illnesses.

Fibromyalgia: Alternate Therapies

Although there is no known cure, you can make some lifestyle changes to manage the symptoms of fibromyalgia.

Exercise

A regular routine of low-impact aerobic activity like swimming, walking, doing yoga, and using cardio machines is widely considered one of the best ways to manage the condition.

Relaxation

Because of the high levels of stress that can accompany fibromyalgia, meditation, yoga, and deep breathing can help.

Cognitive behavioral therapy

Some sufferers find this therapy useful because it offers concrete ways to cope with symptoms.

Acupuncture

Because it works with imbalances in the body, acupuncture along with herbs and moxibustion can help cope with pain.

Bodywork

Feldenkrais, Alexander Technique, and Trager can help alleviate pain by realigning the body and teaching proper body mechanics.

Nutrition

Boost your immune system by eating a healthy diet filled with fruits, vegetables, and whole grains; increase intake of omega-3 fatty acids; eat ginger and turmeric; and take extra magnesium and calcium daily to help relax and maintain nerves and muscles.

Fibromyalgia: Mainstream Therapy

Over-the-counter pain relievers such as Advil, Motrin, or Tylenol

Help with stiffness and pain.

Antidepressants

Help you sleep better and relieve muscle and joint pain.

Muscle relaxants/sleeping pills

Improve sleep.

Menopause

Menopause most commonly happens in a woman's forties and fifties. Marked by an end to the childbearing years, this is when a woman stops having her period and experiences symptoms related to the lack of estrogen production. By definition, a woman is in menopause after her periods have stopped for one year. The drop in estrogen levels triggers all sorts of changes, including hot flashes, night sweats, depression, anxiety, fatigue, weight gain, and decreased sex drive. As with any condition, the severity of the symptoms varies widely.

Menopause: Alternative Approaches

Some people believe that menopause is a natural phenomenon rather than a disease and should be treated naturally. Others feel that the hormonal imbalance interferes with quality of life and should be dealt with through a medical approach. Luckily for today's women, options exist for both extremes.

Acupuncture

Can relieve symptoms like hot flashes, anxiety, insomnia, and irritability by helping the energy move freely.

Acupressure

Brings relief by pressing on the body's meridians and boosting circulation of blood and lymph.

biofeedback relaxation technique

Helps a woman learn to control hot flashes.

Phytoestrogens

Help relieve menopausal symptoms because they are thought to have estrogen-like effects and help relieve hot flashes and night sweats. Try soy products with isoflavones, such as tofu, soy milk, tempeh, and soybeans.

Black cohosh and evening primrose oil

Believed to help hot flashes.

Flaxseed

Also known as linseed; often used to decrease many symptoms of menopause and has been shown to lower breast cancer risk in women.

Dong quai

Supports and maintains the natural balance of female hormones.

Vitamin E

Can help alleviate hot flashes.

B vitamins

May help women deal with the stress of menopausal symptoms.

Menopause: Mainstream Therapy

Reams have been written about the pros and cons of hormone replacement therapy (HRT), and it's emerging as one of the most controversial topics in women's health today. Basically, this treatment supplements the body with either estrogen alone or a combination of estrogen and progesterone to support the hormones no longer adequately produced by a woman's body during menopause.

Some studies show that HRT relieves symptoms like hot flashes and reduces the risk of osteoporosis, hip fractures, and colon cancer. But other studies show an increased risk of breast cancer, stroke, blood clots, and heart disease. To make a decision, it's important to weigh the known risks and benefits, tune in to your body's wisdom, and know that there is no "right" choice.

To break it down, two major kinds of HRT exist: estrogen replacement therapy (ERT), during which estrogen is taken alone, and progestin-estrogen therapy (PET), which combines doses of estrogen and progesterone (progestin is a synthetic form of progesterone). A more detailed description of HRT is beyond the confines of this book; to get more information see your doctor, talk to friends, and do independent research.

Osteoporosis

We've all seen the images of women stooped over and fielded warnings of what will happen if we don't take our calcium: osteoporosis. With this disease, bones lose their mass and become fragile and prone to fracture. Eight million America women and two million American men have osteoporosis, and millions more have low bone density. So how do we know if we are more susceptible? Risk factors include advanced age, family history, absence of periods, and inactive lifestyle.

Three types of osteoporosis exist: Type I happens when estrogen production falls as a result of menopause, and the most common type of bone fractures are vertebral and hip.

Age-associated osteoporosis, or Type II, occurs in both men and women over sixty-five; its primary cause is bone loss due to increased bone turnover over a lifetime. The most common fracture with Type II is hip, as well as the dreaded "dowager's hump." A specific disease causes Type III, or secondary osteoporosis.

Osteoporosis: Alternative Therapies

You can slow the progress of osteoporosis. Protect your bones! The best ways include the following:

Exercise
Do weight-bearing exercises at least four times a week to help keep bones strong and healthy.

Nutrition
Forgo excess carbs, as well as caffeine, alcohol, and sugar.

Calcium
Eat more calcium-rich foods, or take a supplement to maintain healthy bones.

Vitamin D
Take this vitamin to increase calcium absorption, resulting in a reduction of bone loss.

Osteoporosis: Mainstream Approach

Estrogen has been shown to protect women against bone loss. After menopause, estrogen levels drop dramatically, so women rapidly start losing bone mass.

Estrogen replacement therapy

Studies have shown that this therapy cuts fracture rates by at least 50 percent.

Progesterone and testosterone replacement

Helps maintain bone health.

Bisphosphonates

Slow the rate of bone thinning.

Raloxifene (Evista)

Slows bone thinning and increases bone thickness.

Calcitonin (Calcimar or Miacalcin)

Helps regulate calcium levels and relieves pain caused by spinal compression fractures.

Surgery

Vertebroplasty and kyphoplasty, two surgical treatments, may relieve persistent pain from spinal compression fractures resulting from osteoporosis. In these procedures, a surgeon injects bone cement into the crushed spinal bones (vertebrae) through a needle.

Depression

Lethargy. Sadness. Hopelessness. Many of us have experienced these feelings, to varying degrees, throughout our lives. But the majority of those dealing with depression are women; in fact, depression is twice as likely to strike women as men, and from 10 to 25 percent of women will experience an episode of major depression at some time in their lives.[10]

According to the National Institutes of Health, reproductive, genetic, or other biological factors, interpersonal factors, and certain psychological and personality characteristics contribute to the higher levels of depression in women. In addition, women who have experienced some of the following are at a higher risk for depression: loss of a parent before age ten, childhood physical or sexual abuse as a child, mood disorders in early reproductive years or family history of mood disorders, use of certain oral contraceptives or infertility treatments, and ongoing stress factors such as divorce or loss of job.

As you might imagine, depression manifests in different ways for women than for men. For women, depression may occur earlier, last longer, be more likely to recur, be more likely to be associated with stressful life events, and be more sensitive to seasonal changes. Women are more likely to experience guilty feelings and attempt suicide, although they are successful less often than men. Depression in women is more likely to be associated with anxiety disorders, especially panic and phobic symptoms, and eating disorders. Interestingly, depressed women are less likely to abuse alcohol and other drugs.

Depression: Alternative Therapies

These are general guidelines. Because so many kinds of depression exist—chronic, bipolar, seasonal, psychotic, postpartum, to name a few   it's impossible to match exactly what alternative therapy will work best. And remember, many of these haven't been scientifically proven to treat depression.

Herbal supplements

Saint John's wort: Can ease mild to moderate depression.

Ginkgo biloba: Can reduce frequency and intensity of
   depression.

Acupuncture

Can help correct the body's imbalances that lead to depression.

Exercise

*Can help alleviate the symptoms of depression by boosting your
   endorphins.*

Meditation

*Helps you clear your mind and observe your thoughts, bringing about
   a sense of calm and quiet.*

Massage

*Helps to release tension and stored-up emotions and to promote well-
   being, through gentle touching, rubbing, and kneading.*

Guided imagery

*Helps depression by leading you into a state of deep relaxation and
   using the power of your imagination for healing.*

Alternative therapies

Can help to ease depression through self-expression in the arts, movement, and music therapy, leading to a sense of ease in the body and stimulating endorphins.

Yoga

Balances the body's energy centers through poses, breathing exercises, and meditation. Used in combination with other treatment for depression, anxiety, and stress-related disorders.

Biofeedback

Retrains you to deal with anxiety and depression.

Depression: Mainstream Therapies

Psychotherapy

Talking out your problems with a trained professional is often the first step for depression; here, you will get to the underlying issues of your depression, with the goal of gaining a sense of control over your life.

Medications

Can help to improve symptoms of depression by affecting the brain's chemistry. You need to work with a trained doctor to find the best kind for you; medications include tricyclic antidepressants (TCAs), monoamine oxidase inhibitors (MAOIs), and selective serotonin reuptake inhibitors (SSRIs).

What's Your Mindset?

In addition to listening to your body and observing your intuition, carefully examine your mindset. The mind/body connection is a powerful factor in many treatments. Often, the more we believe that a treatment will work, the more likely we are to see results. Many people go into treatments, especially alternative treatments, feeling that they are a last-ditch resort or not believing that they will really work. In your own circumstance, ask yourself if you are open to or skeptical of the treatment. Figure out your opinions, biases, and underlying belief system. Do you believe that psychotherapy is a bunch of baloney? That acupuncture isn't based on sound science? That taking echinacea is a fad? Once you answer these questions, you can then take the most appropriate course of action.

Here are some questions to ask yourself:

→ How much risk do you want to take?

→ To what degree do you believe in the mind/body connection?

→ Are you willing to look at any emotional causes that could exacerbate the condition or illness?

→ Do you trust the practitioner, or do you feel he or she has ulterior motives?

→ Are you open to incorporating lifestyle changes?

→ Are you willing to experiment until you find the right fit?

How to Choose a CAM Practitioner

→ Ask around for referrals from friends and professionals. Find out what conditions each practitioner worked on and if treatment was successful. In addition, ask about the office environment and the practitioner's personality, and find other references.

→ Find out how the practitioner accepts payment. Some won't take insurance; others will work on a sliding scale.

→ Collect information. Do a search on the web, read a book, and arm yourself with knowledge on a particular therapy so you know the right questions to ask.

→ Understand what problems that therapy is most successful in treating.

→ Find out how long the recommended person has been practicing, where he or she was educated, and how many years of school he or she attended.

→ Ask about the practitioner's general philosophy on treatment and care.

→ Trust your instincts. People often try to convince you to do their technique or visit their practitioner. Be polite, but ultimately know that what works for others might not work for you.

Questions to Ask Before Choosing a Complementary or Alternative Treatment:

+ What is the treatment?
+ What does it involve?
+ How does it work?
+ Why does it work?
+ Are there any risks?
+ What are the side effects?
+ Is it effective? (Ask for evidence or proof.)
+ How much does it cost?

Once you answer these questions, discuss the therapy with your doctor. Make sure your doctor knows what therapy you are considering in order to discuss possible interactions with or side effects of your current treatment.

chapter 6

discovering mind/body exercises

Every Tuesday evening throughout my childhood, middle-aged women in leotards and tights appeared at the front door of my suburban home for their weekly yoga class, taught by my mother. They always looked somewhat sheepish when they saw me, as if they were gaining admittance to a slightly off-color event. As yoga teachers went, my mother was the only game in town; she had cobbled together her teaching credentials by going through a series of scattered weekend workshops and by deconstructing hour-long yoga shows on PBS. The ladies padded down the carpeted stairs and into the basement, where they daintily set down their towels and spent the next hour and a half twisting, balancing, bending forward and back, and luxuriating in a final relaxation. They emerged bright eyed and invigorated, chatted for a while, and then headed home to their families.

With my mother leading the pack, these women were my first example of aging gracefully. Even though I didn't know it at the time, their glowing faces, lively gait, and youthful energy proved that aging was actually something to embrace rather than fear. More than two decades later, I find that I have followed in my mother's footsteps. I, too, became a yoga teacher, and I am now instructing students of all ages and health conditions.

One student stands out in my mind. She came to yoga as a "last resort." At forty years old, she was trying to get pregnant, with little luck. Her doctor told her she needed to relax; she had a high-stress job, and to complicate matters, her husband lived a plane ride away. She decided to take some radical measures. Simultaneously, she signed up for acupuncture, chiropractic work, and massage. The first time she came to class, she could barely move her body. She had little body awareness and couldn't keep her eyes closed during the opening and closing meditation. She worked with rugged determination, pushing her body into positions that she wasn't ready for; when I suggested modifications she scoffed. For this high achiever, choosing a modification was a sign of weakness. But the beauty of a mind/body exercise like yoga is that if you keep going back, it eventually works its magic. Sure enough, she began to change. Even though she found many of the poses frustrating, she never missed a class. She began to allow herself to close her eyes during meditation and go within. She loved the time to just sit and breathe. Over time, her body began to unwind; she stopped contorting herself into poses she wasn't ready for and began to take a more relaxed approach to her yoga sessions.

Watching her transformation was magical. It confirmed my belief that the most advanced practice is to go slowly and steadily, respect the body's limitations, and leave your ego aside. In the classes I teach, I always consider the people who take modifications, ease up on a pose, or use a prop not lesser students but yogis who take time to check in with their bodies and see what they need.

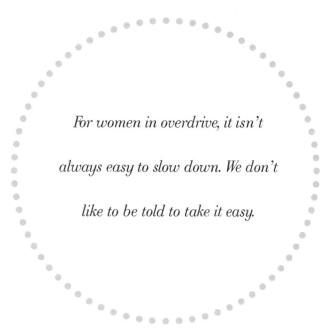

For women in overdrive, it isn't always easy to slow down. We don't like to be told to take it easy.

For women in overdrive, however, this isn't always easy to do. We don't like to be told to take it easy. And if we aren't careful, the very exercises we want to do to calm down, renew, and relax can become causes of major stress when we approach them with an obsessiveness and overly competitive spirit. Not only do we increase the risk of injury, we miss out on big positive returns for our mental and physical well-being.

This is complicated by the fact that as we age, our bodies change. Over time, we can't take the heavy pounding or ultra-high-intensity workouts of the past. If we can't come to grips with the realities of aging and insist on sticking to the routine we did in our twenties, we could be setting ourselves up for long-term injury and a world of pain. Instead, we want to find an exercise where we feel balanced, relaxed—and also physically challenged—and mind/body exercises like yoga and martial arts can hit the right balance for us as we age.

The Mind/Body Connection

"Mind/body" exercises are perfect for women who overdo it—if we work with a sense of consciousness and awareness, instead of just falling into old patterns of striving and achieving above all else. Whereas traditional exercise focuses on an external goal—losing weight, getting six-pack abs, or defining muscle tone—mind/body exercises focus on (you guessed it!) the mind as well as the physical body. Although it's clear the cardiovascular work and muscle strength are important, these exercises also focus on the more subtle effects of exercise. "You don't just train to lose ten pounds; when you train in martial arts it is something that you can incorporate into your whole life," says Bay Area tai chi instructor Mark Wong. In the case of martial arts, the body becomes toned and fit while the mind learns to become calm and relaxed. "You are using that concentration for breathing and moving energy through the body," he explains. Because the form he teaches has a practical application for combat, the "mind" element is crucial: "You have to be calm in combat," he says. "In front of your adversaries, you need to think clearly about how to solve the problem, or if you want to leave the problem."

It's becoming more and more

accepted that the body and

the mind are linked: According

to the American Psychological

Association, 93% of Americans say

that perceptions, thoughts, and

choices affect physical health.

Mind/body exercises engage the person completely in the activity. Think about going to the StairMaster at the gym, where you'll see patrons listening to music on headphones, flipping through magazines, and talking to one another. Instead, a mind/body approach is never about distraction but about connection. Although it still engages the physical body, it's also about connecting with your emotions, your breath, and your activity. So instead of tuning out, we tune in. Taking this one

step further, this kind of engagement can lead to more understanding, respect, confidence, and humility for our world and
ourselves. In other words, we can use these exercises to get
to know ourselves and ask the deeper questions about who
we are and the purpose of our lives, which ultimately leads to
self-actualization.

According to people who work in the fitness field, these
days any mind/body offering they add to the menu blossoms.
And it's becoming more and more accepted that the body and
the mind are linked. According to the American Psychological Association, 93 percent of Americans say that perceptions,
thoughts, and choices affect physical health, while 58 percent
of Americans believe that one can't have good physical health
without good mental health.[1] This shows a profound shift in
popular thinking that moves beyond the increasing numbers
of yogis and martial artists. And it makes sense that women,
often scattered, overworked, and just plain tired, want a place
where they can connect rather than disconnect. Not only does
this make our lives more balanced, but this fuller engagement
also means we're likely to stick with our routines for a longer
period of time and with more enthusiasm.

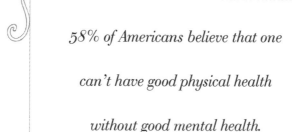

58% of Americans believe that one

can't have good physical health

without good mental health.

Source: American Psychological Association:
www.apahelpcenter.org

Why We Overdo It—and How Not To

This all sounds great, but still, many women simply translate their tendency not to say "enough" into their exercise routines. Overdoing it comes in many forms. For some of us, we feel so much time pressure that it's difficult to simply shift gears. If we are rushing around during the rest of our lives, it makes sense that we will hurry to the gym and rush through our workout without warming up or thinking about what we need for that given day. In our harried culture, we often stop listening to our inner voice. When we can pause and connect to our Self, we can bring back our awareness of that voice. If you are a person who takes classes, you should pay attention to whether your instructor is pointing out the individuality of each person's exercise needs. A good teacher will not tell you to push yourself beyond your limits.

When we are aggressive in our lifestyle, we are aggressive in our exercise. Or if we are very fear driven and overly cautious, this comes out, too. As the Buddhist saying goes, "Not too tight, not too loose." This means that we can approach things in a balanced way. When it comes to exercise, this means that we should avoid injury and unnecessary pain. And it also means that we come to any exercise with a loving attitude about ourselves. One of my favorite writers and teachers, Pema Chödrön, talks about how when we practice, we often work with a "sort of subtle aggression" against who we really are. She writes: "It's a bit like saying, 'If I jog, I'll be a much better person. If I could only get a nicer house, I'd be a better person. If I could meditate and calm down, I'd be a better person.'"[2] The point is to approach exercise to add something to your life, but also to know that you are already okay to begin with, so that if you get injured, ill, or simply unmotivated, you will still have a positive feeling about yourself and who you are. To put it in other words, your identity isn't resting on an external perception of yourself as someone who is fit or thin.

Another tip on not overdoing it? Check your ego at the door. Part of our superwoman status demands that we achieve perfection, don't show weakness, and keep up with the proverbial Joneses. Particularly when we exercise in a group setting, it's tempting to do things we aren't ready for. But when we leave our egos behind, we find that we are doing things only for ourselves and the joy it brings us: that exuberant, radiant feeling that comes after our heart starts pumping and we get into the flow of what we are doing. Even if we learn to ignore the others around us, however, sometimes a more insidious competitor appears —ourselves! Competing with ourselves as we were yesterday, two years ago, or ten years ago is a common occurrence among women in overdrive and one that needs to be taken seriously. Sometimes we don't even realize the endless audiotape inside our heads, telling us we need to *do* more, be more, be better, and perform at a higher level, because that voice has been with us for so long. Part of this process is letting go of that voice.

As I age, I notice that I've started comparing myself to other women more and more. Now that I'm not the youngest—and nowhere near the fittest—one in the room anymore, I am confronted with a new perspective on how I see myself and how others see me. This has been a hard lesson to learn. We want to be the best and the brightest and the most accomplished in the room, something that has been validated since we were young. So it's important to remember that each of us is totally unique. We have different ages, genetics, and physical makeup. Homing in on this idea, and honoring this fact, can help us as we age. Just because someone across the room in your yoga class kicks up into Headstand, you don't have to. In fact, if you aren't ready, you are setting yourself up for injury. I've noticed that I've started thinking more long term in these matters.

The "mind" part of mind/body also means we need to take a more mindful approach to our workouts. With all of the information out there about exercise, diet, aging, and health, we need to educate ourselves and find out what works for us as

individuals. Within our workouts, we can also work with awareness, rather than only effort. This means paying more attention
to our feelings. In yoga, for instance, sometimes you'll feel a
sensation. It's up to you to identify it—is it a burning pain,
which is an indication that a muscle is pulling away from the
bone, or is it a wonderful opening and letting go of tension?
Most of us never pause to have an internal communication with
ourselves, to check in and find out what's really going on.

"When people start stretching, it's uncomfortable, so they
often zone out mentally; they separate their awareness and their
feeling of what they are actually doing," says exercise physiolo-
gist and yoga therapist Meghan Scott. "We need to bring it back
to the internal guidance that tells us that this feels good; you
are safe to open that spot up. And truly, as you know, when you
get into that incredible feeling and everything just opens up,
there is a moment of sheer, ultimate joy."

With all of the information out there

about exercise, diet, aging, and health,

we need to educate ourselves and find

out what works for us as individuals.

I can relate to this feeling. Although I've never been what you might consider a hardcore gym rat, I spent my teens and twenties at the YMCA on the StairMaster, treadmill, and exercise bike. I really dreaded those days; sometimes I'd have a Walkman or a book just so I could get through it. After I started practicing yoga seriously in my late twenties, a whole new world opened up, one where I looked forward to my exercise routine and felt stronger and healthier than I ever had before. Even though I wasn't trying or counting calories, I lost weight and got more muscle tone. And I brought what I learned from my yoga classes into my life—a sense of gentleness, compassion, and the ability to listen to my body and what it needed. I learned that sometimes it's not appropriate to work out; it's sometimes better to stay home, put on some thick socks and sweatpants, and read *People* magazine. This acceptance became okay in my once achievement-oriented exercise obsession. And this helped during my pregnancy, when I became out of breath walking up the stairs and couldn't stroll around the park anymore due to pelvic pain. I learned to take a deep breath and accept this.

Mind/Body Exercises

Any practice can be considered a mind/body exercise if done with conscious awareness. But here are a few that are considered classic mind/body because of their focus on obtaining a meditative state, reducing stress, and moving us toward a deeper understanding of ourselves.

Yoga

What it is: A five-thousand-year-old system of personal
   development that considers the body as a vehicle to unite
   with the divine. Today in America, the main form of yoga
   is composed of the physical poses called hatha yoga, which
   incorporates posture, breath, movement, and meditation.
Who does it: These days? Everyone. That's because you can
   choose from dozens of types of yoga, including iyengar,
   ashtanga, bikram, vinyasa, anusara, viniyoga, and many
   others. Those who are in great shape can do very vigorous
   practice, while those who need a more moderate approach
   can take a gentle class that focuses more on breathing and
   meditating.
What to watch out for: Educate yourself about the type of yoga
   class you want. And once you are there, make sure you find
   the appropriate level. If you are new, take a beginner's class
   to avoid injury. Work at your own pace, and don't compete
   with your neighbor. If you have an injury or illness, find an
   appropriately trained teacher who will help you nurture
   your condition and give you special attention.

Tai Chi

What it is: A slow, repetitive sequence of gentle movements
   created to move the body's energy (called chi), open the
   circulation, relax the muscles, and increase vitality.
Benefits: Helps reverse the physical effects of stress on the
   human body.

Who does it: Those who want a gentle workout, reduced stress, and increased balance and energy.

What to watch out for: If you are expecting a cardiovascular workout, you won't get it here. If you are looking for weight loss or cardiovascular conditioning, incorporate some cardio into your week to complement your tai chi practice.

Qigong

What it is: A Chinese system of physical training, philosophy, and therapeutic healthcare that combines aerobic conditioning, isometrics, isotonics, meditation, and relaxation.

What it does: Improves the delivery of oxygen to the cells, reduces stress, and improves bowel function.

Who does it: Medical qigong is often done by people suffering from many types of disease and illness, including allergies, arthritis, asthma, diabetes, gastritis, gout, headaches, heart disease and hypertension, kidney disease, liver disease, low-back pain, insomnia, substance abuse, ulcers, and chronic pain.

What to watch out for: If you suffer from an illness, stay informed. Don't rely solely on medical qigong; get a variety of assessments and viewpoints first.

Choose Your Path

If you look at the shelves of any bookstore, there are hundreds of books by "experts" on everything from buying real estate to getting six-pack abs to redoing the plumbing in your bathroom. During my pregnancy, I have leafed through books and magazines that dispense advice on sleeping, nursing, parenting, birthing, and every other topic. Each book acts as if it contains the answer. But I believe that we need to follow our intuition when it comes to pregnancy, parenting, exercise, and everything else. So although it runs counter to an "advice" book, we need to listen to our bodies when it comes to choosing an exercise path. Every person has a different exercise threshold. Since some people's bodies can handle more physical stress than others', it's important to start small when choosing an exercise program. Here's how to determine the right exercise for you—but remember that these are only guidelines.

Assess Your Exercise Likes and Dislikes

We are more likely to stick with something we love rather than something we dread. Ask yourself the following questions: Do I like being indoors or outdoors? Do I like exercising alone or in a class setting? Do I like loud music or silence? Would I prefer to be with only other women or in a coed group? These things matter and can help narrow down your choices.

Determine Your Level of Fitness

Get yourself out of a one-size-fits-all mode of thinking. Remember that you might not be able to pick up your old exercise routine after ten years. Or you might not be able to join your best friend as she trains for a marathon. Are you trying to heal an injury? Do you have specific physical limitations, like bad knees, that will determine what you choose?

Take a Crash Course

Educate yourself about fitness—or meet with someone like a personal trainer who can help you. Understand the difference between aerobic exercise, strength, and flexibility, and determine what you want to get out of your workout. "When people come in, if they have very little awareness about their physicality, they will have a very low level of awareness of how their body wants to move," says Jim Karanas, Club One's group fitness director.

Try Everything

Cast a wide net when it comes to exercise. Even something you tried and didn't like several years ago, like weight training or salsa, may appeal to you this time around. New classes keep popping up every day. Take an adventurous approach and have an open mind.

Start Small

To avoid a "crash and burn" approach, whatever you choose to try, start on a small scale. Take a beginner's class rather than an advanced class. Get individual attention or a personal trainer if you have specific injuries or concerns. Start with a modest number of minutes, like twenty, and work your way up.

Think Long Term

You want to find something that you will stick with and something that won't be so hard on your body that you won't be able to continue over time. Talk to a personal trainer about the exercise you choose; he or she can help you craft a routine that's right for you.

Be Gentle

Sometimes less is more. My mother teaches yoga to a couple once a week. They work hard all day and just want to stretch a little and relax. She teaches them chair yoga. "They have stamina, but when they come here they don't want a lot. They swear it helps them all week," she says.

Stay Motivated

Like so many other things we need to fit into our daily lives, exercise can become a dreaded obligation. But staying fully engaged and interested in an exercise program should take top priority in our lives.

For some of us, the joy of feeling energized and revitalized is enough to keep us excited about our exercise regime. It helps, of course, when we find something that we absolutely love to do. When you find something that brings you so much joy, it's hard to feel that same sense of obligation we feel when we have to, say, pay the bills. But a sense of discipline does come into play. Often, we have to talk ourselves into getting there. Ask yourself what will help you stay motivated—and be brutally honest with your answer.

Find Variety

Not only is variety good for your mind, it's good for your body not to repeat the same movements for decades upon decades.

Say No to Peer Pressure

Remember that what works for your best friend, mother-in-law, or coworker may not work for you. Again, each of us has a different constitution and comfort level. So even if another person swears by a certain exercise, remember that you might not like it. And just because your best friend, mother-in-law, or coworker pressures you to keep coming back, that doesn't mean you have to. Quiet down and see what feels right for you.

Before You Start

Understand Your Equipment

"Before you can develop a level of comfort in your body, you must learn the basics," says Karanas. He recommends learning how to use the equipment you'll be working with, for example, how to use the heart rate monitor correctly or how the bike gets different results than the elliptical trainer.

Choose a Focus

Want to improve your cardio capacity? Go for spinning. Looking for more flexibility? Yoga might be for you. Figure out what you want to work on most and go for it.

Go with What Feels Good

Throw the "shoulds" out the window. This is a time for you to enjoy what you do.

Don't just go for the most convenient; go for what you love. This could be kickboxing, Pilates, yoga, or anything else. Try to see how your body likes to move.

Changes as We Age

It's no secret that our bodies change as we age and go through pregnancies, menopause, injuries, and hormonal shifts. My mother is an example of how our exercise routines change over time—and of how we can easily fall into the overdrive trap when it comes to our workouts. She has always been active, and she's tried everything—running, weight lifting, and even going for a short stint to Curves.

She told me, "I wouldn't say I'm a natural exerciser. It's important—I'm health conscious, I want my body to be okay, but I'm not driven and don't feel crazy if I don't do it."

Her main source of exercise has been walking, either on a treadmill or outside. She has been doing yoga since her late twenties. "I loved stretching; it really refreshed me," she says. When she turned sixty-one, however, she began to notice a few changes in her body. Her lower body sometimes hurt after she practiced. "But I just kept pushing," she says, a typical reaction from a woman in overdrive. "I didn't want to stop because I liked it, so I thought I could push my body like before." Like many of us, she had the idea that "more is better." She says, "I just felt that it's so good for me and I wanted to keep limber and keep my figure, but I think I overdid it because I don't notice."

She sustained a sacrum injury that took a year to heal, and then this negatively affected her psoas and piriformis. "It took me a long time to stop doing what I shouldn't do," she says. "I felt I was addicted to stretching. My ligaments were over-stretched, and my bones started moving too much because the ligaments wouldn't hold the bones in place."

Finally she realized that she had to make a change. She cut down on her yoga and began to do tai chi, which at first she didn't like because she felt it was too slow. She also incorporated weight training because she knew it would be good for her. With the help of a trainer at the gym, she learned some simple exercises to help strengthen her body.

The changes haven't been easy for her. "My body gets injured faster; it takes longer to heal. It's hard to accept, very hard." She says recognizing her limitations has been a major test. When I asked her if she would do anything differently if she had the chance, she said she would be smarter about how she exercises, understanding that more isn't always better. She also says she would warm up more frequently and not force her movements if they didn't feel right.

"So now, at sixty-four, I'm concentrating on tai chi, which is easy on the bones and ligaments and more of an internal thing. Other people who do it have had such benefits. It's a proven thing. I still walk. I tire more easily. If I do a lot of walking, it's hard to do a full session of tai chi."

Exercise and Aging: Tips from a Pro

So what are the golden rules to follow when it comes to aging and exercising? "I constantly attest to the fact that I will be fifty-two in January, and I am fitter, leaner, stronger, and faster than when I was twenty," says Karanas. He gave me the following tips:

Integrate Exercise Daily

Instead of considering it a chore, make exercise a daily and continuous event that you engage in time and time again. Work it into your life, whether it's biking to work, walking on your lunch hour, or going on a yoga vacation.

Connect with a Group

It's easier with help. Join a walking group, outdoor cycling program, or cycling club for support and camaraderie.

Support a Cause

What better motivation than to have your exercise help someone else! Walk for AIDS or leukemia, or volunteer for a charitable event to make it possible. "When you are willing to step up and help, giving back and attaching to something that's important makes you feel younger," says Karanas.

Eat Well

Sounds commonsensical, but we all need a gentle reminder every now and then.

Go for Intensity

Years ago, a low level of intensity was recommended for aerobic capacity. Things have changed, according to Karanas. "Training is being somewhat scrutinized," he says. In light of new research on exercise and aging, as we get older we have to work near peak levels of intensity. "We have to create more power as we get older. That's how we start to see so many people in their fifties who are now stronger than when they were twenty," he adds. So challenge yourself and continue to take on challenges as you age.

Take Time to Recover

Research also shows the importance of recovery. Instead of simply taking a day or two off, we need to focus on various types of training that promote "active recovery." For example, if you are an avid biker, this might mean you take a month to stop biking and do restorative yoga. Karanas sees a lot of resis-tance to this idea, because people feel as if they will get out of shape or lose what they've gained in terms of strength. But the experts disagree. "Most people haven't learned the importance of active recovery," says Karanas. "It takes a certain amount of time. Your body needs to retune and restore itself."

The Next Wave

We are always learning new things from science about exercise. Exercise physiologists are constantly measuring ways to achieve optimal fitness: the intervals of aerobic versus slow conditioning, the time it takes to stretch a muscle to its maximum. With this in mind, the next wave of exercise includes an awareness of the consciousness behind fitness. As a society, we are tired of working just to lose weight or gain muscle. More fundamentally, we are starting to think about the consciousness behind fitness.

Jim Karanas sees this trend at the twenty Club One fitness clubs he oversees. He observes overwhelming interest in classes that help "develop you as a person," rather than classes focused solely on burning calories. "When people are engaged just on a physical level, the adherence is very bad," he says. "They will tend to put exercise off and think, *I just have one more thing to do.* But when a training system engages people more, as a system of self-development of both body and soul, it's not something that can be put aside, and that modality becomes very important to you and you can return to it when things go sideways in your life." He says step and aerobics classes are examples of classes that don't engage a person. He says that although step is a good training system for the body, there is "everything wrong with it. It's too fast and too complex. You can't really connect a philosophy with it. People will get bored because there is nothing deeper." He points to modalities like biking and running as examples of great training systems that also have a deep meditative and philosophical level to them. Even at the mainstream gyms, Karanas sees the overall popularity of holistic health on the rise. "It's not just in health clubs," he says. "If you look at society as a whole, we are going more toward a wellness mindset."

Karanas also warns that some systems, like yoga and spinning, started out as conscious exercises, but beware of those classes that have been "bastardized" by Western culture. He uses the examples of karaoke spinning classes and hot yoga, both of which take the traditional form and twist it around with an external focus, losing the original intention.

So what's next on the exercise horizon? "We are going to start seeing a lot of fusion classes growing out of the fact that right now, the over-fifty-five group is the fastest-growing group and the second-fastest-growing group is under eighteen," says Karanas. This means that the over-fifty-five group has grown tired of its usual routine and is eager to learn something new, like salsa or belly dancing. And because of the demand for these classes, the under-eighteen crowd will be exposed to them as well. Here are a few of the ways health clubs and gyms are getting creative with the idea of group exercise, either by creating hybrids or by finding new ways to get the body moving.

Hot for Hybrids

A few popular fusion classes are popping up at health clubs across the country:

Bhangra Dance

One of India's most popular folk dances, bhangra involves a high-energy yet soulful workout that is done to the sounds of an Indian drum.

Yogalates

A mixture of yoga and Pilates.

Bosulates

A hybrid of Bosu (which stands for "both sides up" and uses an exercise ball that's been cut in half, with a platform on the bottom) and Pilates.

Nia

Short for "neuromuscular integrative action," Nia fuses elements from dance, martial arts, and healing arts to encourage a sense of freedom through conscious and gentle movement.

Capoeira

A form of Afro-Brazilian martial arts that emphasizes endurance and strength.

Cycle Karaoke

You guessed it. Sing while you ride.

Masala Bhangra

The traditional Indian dance workout set to hip-hop, disco, salsa, techno, house, and rap music.

Ballet Boot Camp

Strength-building exercises combined with ballet moves.

Dembo

A combination of dance and aerobics using Latin, Indian, and Arabic moves.

Yoga Ballet

A fusion of yoga and ballet.

Vindalini Yoga

Unites two kinds of yoga: a flow-based vinyasa and the more meditative kundalini practice.

Yogic Arts

A fusion of ashtanga and the elements of Kuk Sool Sun martial arts.

Mind/Body as Medicine

Holistic approaches have a saying: "Your issues are in your tissues." I've always loved this idea, which is really saying that our emotions are a body-based experience. We hold joys, hurts, and traumas on a cellular level in our bodies. Studies have shown that we have as much nervous tissue in our bellies as in our brains, which is one reason why exercises like yoga make us feel better, because they remove energetic blocks and get our life force going. When we block or suppress emotions, we often experience physical symptoms. A whole sector of neuroscience has emerged to study this phenomenon: Traumatic experiences get stored, and our neuropeptide receptor sites shrink in size and get dull and blocked, according to Richard Faulds, a senior teacher at Kripalu Center for Yoga & Health in Lenox, Massachusetts. "The bottom line is that powerful experiences that we cannot fully digest or integrate somehow get stored in the actual tissues of our body and they block our vitality," he says. At Kripalu, Faulds sees visitors with unresolved emotional baggage (which he also calls body armor, repression, and suppression of powerful emotions) suffering from three levels of physical symptoms: The first level includes chronic neck or back pain, migraine headaches, chronic fatigue, insomnia, and low immune response. The second level is anxiety attacks, panic attacks, and depression. And the last level is serious illness and disease.

We can see why it's important to focus on both the mind and the body and how each one supports the other. David Simon is the cofounder and medical director of the Chopra Center for Wellbeing at the La Costa Resort & Spa in Carlsbad, California. "We know there is this intimate mind/body relationship," he says. "Where internal dialogue is of regret, for instance, that actually translates into weakened immune function, and you are more susceptible to everything from colds to cancer. On every level we find it helpful for people to identify what emotions they haven't fully digested and the mind is so good at suppressing. It's important to do something liberating to release them and commit yourself to new choices and start cultivating nourishment in our lives."

restoring the body during sickness and disease

I've been surrounded by women who do too much. My grand-mother Frances suffered from many physical problems that required her to rely on others yet looked upon asking for help as somehow shameful. My mother tends to overdo it and often tires herself out by expending huge amounts of energy when she's already depleted. It's not uncommon for her to need the next day to recover. My first writing mentor worked at a high-stress magazine-editing job and took pride in her constant state of incredible productivity at work, coming in at the crack of dawn and staying late while also managing to cook gourmet meals for her family every night.

So while I admire these women deeply for their love of life, generosity, dedication to family, and compassion, it's no wonder that I've internalized equating success with overdoing it. Most of the women in my life feel overwhelmed with work, family responsibilities, relationships, and the simple care of the basics. In my own life, my pregnancy has limited my work life, social engagements, and physical prowess. But even when I know I should nap instead of meeting a friend for tea, turn down an assignment that has a one-week turnaround, or even walk more slowly up the stairs, it takes a conscious effort to stop my mind from convincing me otherwise. Overdoing it has become commonplace for us women, and even expected. Some of us, in fact, take a certain pride in overdoing it, a badge of honor that elevates us above the fray of those who simply can't handle anything and everything thrown their way. It becomes our identity, a mark of superiority to counter the outdated idea that women are fragile creatures, swooning in the heat or suffering from nervous conditions that require us to sit in our rooms and stare at the wallpaper.

In 1950, about 1 in 3 women participated in the labor force. By 1998, nearly 3 of every 5 women of working age were in the labor force. Among women age 16 and over, the labor force participation rate was 33.9% in 1950, compared with 59.8% in 1998.

Source: Department of Labor Statistics:
www.bls.gov/opub/

Of course, times have changed. In 1950, about one in three women participated in the labor force. By 1998, nearly three of every five women of working age were in the labor force. Among women age sixteen and over, the labor force participation rate was 33.9 percent in 1950, compared with 59.8 percent in 1998.[1] We are earning more money, gaining higher job status, working longer hours, and taking on more responsibilities—but we don't necessarily adjust the rest of our lives to accommodate these things. Without a kind of escape valve for our stress and feelings of being overwhelmed, the result is a constant state of overdrive. If we aren't careful, our health suffers as we age in ways both big and small.

Overdoing it has become commonplace for us women, and even expected. Some of us, in fact, take a certain pride in overdoing it, a badge of honor that elevates us above the fray of those who simply can't handle anything and everything thrown their way. It becomes our identity, a mark of superiority to counter the outdated idea that women are fragile creatures, swooning in the heat or suffering from nervous conditions that require us to sit in our rooms and stare at the wallpaper.

Well past our twenties—when we didn't think too much about our health and longevity—we still don't connect the dots between overdoing it and becoming ill. In fact, many women don't slow down until we get the news that most of us thought we would never get, news that we dread: that we have a disease.

For Zoe Elton, a film festival programming director, that meant a diagnosis of breast cancer. For Susan Dubrof, who has multiple sclerosis, this translated as ignoring the detrimental effects of her stressful, eighty-hour workweek as an attorney. My guess is that millions of other women faced with both sudden disease and chronic illness would point to a state of constant overdrive as a prime culprit in their condition. By no means am I placing any blame on the person who gets sick. Rather, I'm reflecting what many women have told me—that they don't realize, or don't let sink in, how much their stressful existence affects their health.

"Stress was a primary, primary cause," says Zoe of her disease. "When I was diagnosed, I immediately understood that in a sort of metaphorical way. As the treatment evolved, I got tangible responses that told me that what I had been doing in terms of my working life had compromised my immune system. I feel like I've been complicit in this."

Without a kind of escape

valve for our stress and feelings

of being overwhelmed, the result is

a constant state of overdrive.

Zoe: Coping with Breast Cancer

Zoe Elton, a vibrant redhead, was advised to get a second set of photographs and a sonogram after a routine mammogram. "I knew it didn't look good," says Zoe. But she realized the seriousness of her results when the nurse asked, "Do you have anyone with you?"

"When I got the diagnosis, I went into this really odd, focused kind of place," says Zoe. "I really got to understand the notion of living in the moment. Before it was something that you just kind of hear. You just get completely plunged into the fire. Anything that existed before doesn't exist," Zoe adds. And she isn't the only one dealing with this news: Over the past fifty years, breast cancer has increased each year, and today approximately one in almost every eight women (13.4 percent) will develop the disease. It's the second leading cause of cancer death in women after lung cancer—and is the leading cause of cancer death among women ages thirty-five to fifty-four.[2]

At the time of her diagnosis, Zoe worked between sixty and eighty hours a week. "It became obsessive; it became consuming," she says of her job, which took her around the world to film festivals, in addition to her regular work schedule. "There was always more. I was incapable of saying no, and that really damaged a lot of areas—my social life and my family life. When your friends call you and everything they say is prefaced by, 'I know you are busy but . . .' it's not good."

Over the past 50 years, breast

cancer has increased each year,

and today approximately 1 in

almost every 8 women (13.4%) will

develop the disease. It's the second

leading cause of cancer death in

women after lung cancer—and is

the leading cause of cancer death

among women ages 35 to 54.

Source: www.webmd.com/content/

When she got her diagnosis, Zoe was forced to confront what lay at the heart of her untenable work schedule. Finally, she had to deal with the part of her life she had been avoiding. For Zoe, the root of losing herself in an all-consuming job was grief. Over a very short period of time, she had experienced the death of both of her parents, the death of several friends to AIDS, and the end of a ten-year relationship.

"What happened was just so cumulative," she recalls. "I thought I was having a bad year, but it turned into a bad few years. It was relentless. I didn't see a therapist, I didn't see anybody, and I kept soldiering on —and failing at everything."

It's this very idea of "soldiering on" that strikes a chord with so many ambitious, driven, and determined women. It makes us feel strong and powerful, perhaps. Or maybe we don't see any other options ahead of us. In thinking about the metaphor, it's almost violent. A soldier is someone who fights in a battle, and the phrase implies that our lives are like battles that need to be fought and won. This analogy aptly describes many women who feel as if they have to fight tooth and nail to get ahead of their game at the expense of everything that's important, like their health.

For many of us, this is tied into our changing roles as women, especially when it comes to work. My husband, for example, has no trouble setting boundaries with his coworkers, saying no to projects he doesn't have time to complete, and communicating directly with his boss. On the other hand, these are the issues that I've struggled with over my entire career.

But eventually, we find that we just can't soldier on any longer. Whether we are confronted with this fact because of illness, divorce, midlife crisis, or a total reevaluation of our lives, it doesn't matter. If we want to be healthy and prioritize what's important in our lives, we have to agree to surrender some of the time.

Susan: Dealing with Multiple Sclerosis

Susan Dubrof, who was diagnosed with MS in 1985, says that she was in denial about the fact that stress caused her any difficulty. With a nagging feeling that changing her life and work habits would be "giving in" to her disease, she justified her high levels of stress in order to maintain her life—despite the progression of her illness.

Susan often experienced exacerbations of her symptoms but denied any links between her levels of stress and these incidences. "Being the social scientist I am, I had great store in the fact that there had been no *definitive* studies directly linking exacerbations or lesions or progression of the illness with stress. Never mind the fact that I hadn't looked at the few studies out there that *do* try to look at that. I just accepted the conclusion."

She remembers one day when another woman with MS told Susan that she had slowed the progression of her illness by retiring. "This was disturbing to me," Susan recalls. "I didn't want to stop working, and I talked myself into the belief that work was a kind of positive stress."

But on some level, Susan knew better.

Looking back, she realizes that her refusal to see the connection was just a psychological effort to protect herself from the reality of her situation—that she was living with a degenerative disease that made her different from the people around her. In order to come to grips with this, she entered into therapy, where she says she learned to examine the things she doesn't like about herself.

Susan's reaction to her illness makes perfect sense when you consider that she's spent a lifetime as an overachiever. As a child, she skipped two grades. She attended Yale and always held prestigious positions. After her diagnosis, she opted for the high-stress world of law school. "My diagnosis kind of propelled me to do something I had always said I'd do. I thought, *Better do this sooner than later.*" She graduated from law school and went to work as a labor lawyer, where she worked long hours to bring in money for the firm. As the laws in Oregon changed, to the detriment of injured workers, her job got harder and harder.

"In 1998, I had four flare ups, which is really a lot. I was having trouble bringing enough income." During one month, she took only one day off. Finally she realized she needed to make a change. First, she cut down her hours to forty a week, after which she witnessed a dramatic decrease in her income. She soon decided to leave private practice and started working for the City of Portland. "I started acknowledging the stress and doing something about it," she says. Indeed, she couldn't ignore it anymore: In 2000, walking became so difficult that she got fitted for a brace on her right leg. A year later, she got a brace for her left leg, and her doctor recommended a scooter for long distances. Perhaps even more traumatic for this Ivy League alumna was a neuropsychological exam that produced distressing results. "I was face to face with not being able to complete these tests."

Another turning point happened soon after a big flare-up of Susan's symptoms. Her doctor recommended rehabilitation, but a day before she was scheduled to start, she went into a state of panic and rushed herself to the ER, thinking she was dying because she couldn't breathe well. But the tests showed nothing. "As soon as I was tucked in, I asked my nurse if she was going to take care of me. When she said yes, it was like this curtain lifting. Because of anxiety, I had convinced myself that I couldn't breathe and that I was dying. I had never realized what my mind was capable of doing to me. I couldn't deal with the realities of this illness and needed to do something other than denying it and pushing through."

Pushing through, soldiering on. Variations on this theme resonate throughout a woman's life as she ages. When it comes to a critical juncture, women like Zoe and Susan have a choice: They can either use the situation as a wake-up call, or they can just push through and then get back to business as usual. Not all of us experience such dramatic turning points, but it's worthwhile to stop and examine this notion. As caretakers, who will take care of us when we need it—not just when we find ourselves in life-threatening situations, but on a day-to-day basis? Self-sufficiency has its place, but it's necessary to find a balance between self-sufficiency and self-destruction. Maybe it's just realizing that we can't have a home-cooked meal every night for our family, or that we need to ask our partner to clean the bathroom once in a while. Maybe it's understanding that it's all right to ask a friend to bring over some soup when you aren't feeling so great, or that you need to allocate the money you spend on cable for a housecleaner instead. Little things like these can quite possibly avert a "big thing" from happening by making us feel supported, safe, and comforted.

As for Susan, she finally decided to stop working altogether. It was only then she realized just how stressful her life had become. "I just couldn't believe what it was like to actually be rested for the first time, and to not beat my head against the wall regarding work that I could no longer do as quickly, and had grown to kind of hate."

It Takes a Village

The overachievers among us like to think of ourselves as über-competent, cool, and capable. Indeed, we women don't often ask for help. I notice that I have a difficult time with this, even among my closest friends. A sense of guilt comes over me; *they are too busy, too tired, too preoccupied with their own lives,* I think. I don't want them to go out of their way or disturb their routine. I think I should perhaps wait until I *really* need a big favor so I don't ask for too much over time. Ironically, helping my friends is one of the great pleasures of my life, so it's interesting I still have that ingrained attitude. But when faced with an illness, asking for help is often the first time we allow ourselves to be vulnerable enough to really embrace something that is actually a valuable skill.

"When dealing with the stress of a very serious illness, it brings an incredible lucidity, and you really strip away from any excesses of things that you don't need in your life—people and everything else," says Zoe.

First, Zoe needed to deal with her diagnosis on her own. When she got home from the hospital after hearing the news, she immediately called another friend with breast cancer. But she didn't get through, a serendipitous fact when she looks back on it. "I realized that calling her wasn't the right thing to do. I needed to deal with my situation." After she spent some time processing the illness on her own, she decided to tell only one person at work and a few close friends. "I chose people who I could relate to both personally and spiritually. That was pretty important to me."

As time went on, Zoe found that she needed to assemble a team of people who would understand and support her. She thought about going to a support group but ended up not going. She found it too depressing. "I didn't want to hear any bad stories; it doesn't help," she says. She went to a few yoga classes for people with cancer, but that didn't work out, either. "I just felt like everybody else was so much sicker than me." She ended up finding support from people she already knew—friends and peers who had things in common with her, people with similar backgrounds, people of a like mind.

She was surprised at the challenge of giving people the news. "There's something odd about telling people you have cancer," she says. "It's very intimate; I didn't realize it beforehand, but it's almost shameful. I don't know if it's my particular upbringing, but it feels like a failure. Your body is failing."

Zoe's disclosure reminds me of an experience I had when I attended a yoga retreat at Esalen, a beautiful and expansive retreat center located along the rugged coast of Big Sur. I fainted during one of my yoga classes. I simply passed out. Before I hit the floor, though, I grabbed the woman next to me for some support as I went down. When I awoke, I experienced that same feeling of failure that Zoe describes. I had tried to keep up with everybody in the class, although I was the only pregnant person in the room. I wanted to just be normal, be like everybody else. Still, my plan backfired.

Why did I feel ashamed at fainting? This ingrained sense of failure at not living up to expectations comes from a deep place. As I lay on the ground, I realized that it's within my power to feel shame or not. So I surrendered to the fact that I fainted. I let the strangers in the class put me gently down on a blanket, call the nurse, and sit with me for a while. I made a conscious effort to *not* feel guilty for disrupting the class and just tried to accept the fact this was happening. And let me tell you, it felt good.

Tuning in to Your Body

Many women are totally blindsided by their diagnoses, while others knew that something was wrong all along. Zoe remembers thinking to herself often, *I know I need to change things, but what would I do if I got cancer?* At that point, she says, she probably already realized on some level that she had a lump. In fact, when her boss asked her to travel to Berlin, she told him she

couldn't go because she would be having some health problems. "I could almost see the words coming out of my mouth,
like a talk bubble," she says.

Interestingly, Zoe says, once she came home with the diagnosis, the signs she had been ignoring were not all that subtle.
Someone had given her *Anatomy of the Spirit,* by Caroline Myss,
a healing intuitive, and she had bookmarked a chapter talking
about the importance of making a vow to yourself to do everything you can do to heal emotionally, spiritually, and physically. "I walked out of the hospital and into a vow," says Zoe. "I
thought, *Okay, I'm hearing you.* That's what I had to do."

Once they slow down, women in overdrive, like Zoe and
Susan, often turn to alternative approaches to healing their
minds and bodies. And this is an increasingly growing trend.
Hospitals and wellness centers that specialize in everything
from heart problems and cancer to too much stress and other
ailments are now incorporating yoga, meditation, deep breathing, guided imagery, and visualization into their programs for
a more holistic and integrative approach to strengthening the
body, focusing the mind, and bouncing back from disease.

Alternative Approaches to Healing: Yoga

For Susan, her yoga practice was a continuation of something she had started more than twenty years before. Always athletic, she found that yoga introduced her to something totally new. "I never had a way to consciously relax," she says.

As her illness progressed, she found it increasingly difficult to attend her classes. In 1997, she attended a yoga class at the MS Society that modified the poses—something she didn't even know was possible. In addition to finding help for her range of motion and increasingly contracted muscles, she found something deeper: "I was encouraged to look inside, a place I was always racing away from, and so yoga really coincided so much with just what I emotionally needed."

After Zoe's lymph node surgery and six weeks of radiation, she couldn't move her arm and ultimately got a frozen shoulder. Her condition got worse and worse. So she started doing a small yoga practice every day and has kept it up. Now that her strength is up, she sometimes goes to hour-long classes at a local studio. Even this represents a major shift in her thinking. In the past, her thinking was, *I'd like to go to the class, but I've got more work to do.* Now, she says, the yoga habit is so embedded in her life that she prioritizes it. And she includes breathwork in her routine. "I kept thinking about the breath after my diagnosis, I think partly because when you are told you have a cancer, you are facing death," she says. "It made me think about seeing both my mom and dad die, and seeing them take their last breaths."

A Calming Breath

This simple exercise can be done anytime, anyplace. Find a comfortable cross-legged position and close your eyes. Bring your awareness to your breath, and notice its quality. Is it deep or shallow? Do you have long or short inhalations and exhalations? Once you've noticed, then try to make the breath as long and as smooth as possible. Place your left hand on your belly and your right hand on your chest. As you inhale, feel your belly rise and your chest rise. As you exhale, feel your chest fall and your abdomen pull slightly in. With each breath, imagine that you are filling your lungs to the very top and then squeezing all of the air out of the lungs. If you feel dizzy, return the breath to normal. Continue this deep abdominal breathing for five minutes. Then slowly release your hands to your thighs or knees and return your breath to normal.

Meditation

Both Susan and Zoe found meditation an invaluable tool in their healing process. "I already had a meditation practice. That was huge, absolutely huge. I'm just very, very grateful that was already in place," says Zoe. She thinks back to her life years ago, before she established a meditation practice, and sees how she reacts differently to the stresses in her life. "It brings you back to working on a cellular level," she says. "I think between a meditation practice and doing stuff with kids, my body was able to deal better, in terms of engaging with the illness."

Susan also credits a deepened meditation with helping move from denial to acceptance of her illness. "It's helped me understand that pain is part of life, but suffering is something that we have some control over— and that is so freeing. Meditation has given me this way to be with my fearful, crazed, angry, sorry, sad, happy, loving self and realize that they are just feelings and they aren't going to kill me They come and go. I didn't ever learn as a young person to soothe myself or have my feelings. I learned a way of surviving by pretty much denying my feelings. In my family, there wasn't a quality of compassion— there was love that wasn't expressed. It was pretty rough on everybody."

As Susan learned, a meditation practice can help to cultivate a sense of compassion toward ourselves. And we can do that in a safe place—on a mat. Once we can learn to return to the breath and gently bring the wandering mind

Vipassana Meditation

Buddhists refer to the thinking mind as a "monkey mind" because it jumps around just like a monkey scrambling from one branch to the next. But you can't tame the monkey in meditation by just sitting down and trying your very best not to think. Vipassana, a form of meditation taught by the Buddha more than 2,500 years ago, gives some guidelines on how to deal with the endless stream of thoughts we experience. Also called "insight meditation," vipassana helps you observe your thoughts and ultimately gain insight into them. As you start to understand how your mind operates, you will eventually notice yourself developing more wisdom, clarity, and compassion. Here is how to do it:

Sit in a straight-back position, with your arms resting comfortably on your knees. Close your eyes. Scan your body for tension, and if you find any, consciously relax that area. Next, place your

attention on your breath where it enters and leaves your nostrils. When your mind wanders from your breath, notice where it is going and silently label this. If you find you are planning, say, what to make for dinner, silently say, "Planning, planning" to yourself, watch as the thought dissolves, and then return your attention to your breath. If you notice you want something different from what's happening in the present moment, label it "Grasping." If you feel anger or fear, silently say, "Aversion." If your eyelids start to droop, say to yourself, "Sleepiness." Continue in this way, each time labeling your thoughts as they arise and then watching them, without judgment, as they dissipate. Beginners can try this for five minutes, and more advanced meditators can do it for half an hour. When you are done, slowly open your eyes and take a few deep breaths into your abdomen before getting up.

back from wherever it meanders—and do so without judging ourselves—the seeds are planted: We learn compassion.

"Compassion is everything, in terms of accepting the world as it is," says Susan. "It has helped me so much with my MS. Now I am willing to face it in all that it means and all that it requires of me, which is really just taking care of me. It's just a revelation."

Imagery

When Zoe had her first surgery, a friend helped her with some visualization the night before her lumpectomy. Over the phone, her friend helped her imagine her spirit returning back to her body after the surgery. Zoe also decided that she needed to personify her tumors. She called them "the gossips" and decided that they were there to teach her something. So she started to talk to them, even thanking them for coming and putting the issues she was avoiding on the table. "I wanted to have an image of accepting that they were there, and then asking them to leave and promising that I would work on the issues that they were there to deal with."

Guided imagery—using the power of the imagination to help the healing process—has gained traction across the country. In fact, a growing body of research on guided imagery shows its effectiveness for dozens of conditions that involve high levels of stress, including anxiety, chemotherapy, cardiac surgery, pain, depression, diabetes, irritable bowel syndrome, and anxiety before MRIs and radiation.

A turning point for imagery occurred in the late nineties, with research that revolved around surgery: Time after time, studies showed that pre- and post-surgery patients who used imagery had a shorter average hospital stay, experienced a decrease in pain and anxiety, and used fewer drugs. A few years later, a much-referenced Blue Shield of California study done with hysterectomy patients again showed shorter stays, less pain, and a dramatic decrease in anxiety, but also another important finding: Those who used imagery reduced the insurance company's bill by 14 percent.[3]

Cumulatively, these studies led to a greater awareness, which led to the hundreds of studies being conducted today in areas that go far beyond pre-surgery patients. The most comprehensive studies concern anxiety, pain management, and oncology, but research has been conducted on allergies, menopause, hypertension, carpal tunnel syndrome, geriatric insomnia, herpes, and others.

Beyond the hard facts, experts say imagery plays a crucial role in a medical setting by empowering people to take charge of their health. Instead of being prodded by doctors and told what to do, women who use imagery can feel a sense of participating in their own healing.

Attitude

Every person deals with disease in different ways. Some ask, "Why me?" Others deny the severity of their condition. Some withdraw, and others reach out. Some plunge headfirst into the medical community, and others look for alternative ways of healing. Whatever women choose, they all seem to find that attitude is a key factor in their progress.

Metta Meditation

You can't love anybody else if you don't love yourself first. That is the premise of metta meditation, a Buddhist form that encourages an openhearted nurturing of yourself and others, imperfections and all. *Metta*, the Pali word for lovingkindness, helps to cultivate feelings of love and acceptance through a systematic repetition of phrases. Try these simple steps.

Sit comfortably and take a few deep breaths into the belly. Silently offer metta to yourself: *May I be safe. May I be healthy. May I be joyful. May I be free.* Stop after each phrase, take a deep breath, and notice how it feels to wish yourself well. After a few minutes, start to extend these wishes outward: Think of someone you love deeply. With that person in mind, silently repeat: *May she be safe. May she be healthy. May she be joyful. May she be free.*

After a few moments, think of a "neutral" person, someone you see on the bus or behind the coffee counter. Repeat the phrases with her in mind. Then think of someone you have a difficult relationship with. Silently repeat the metta meditation toward that person. Finally, extend metta out to all beings everywhere. *May all beings be safe. May all beings be healthy. May all beings be joyful. May all beings be free.* As you start to become familiar with the phrases, feel free to change the words around so that they resonate with you completely; some people even like to put them to a melody. When you are done with your metta session, take a few deep breaths, bring your hands to your heart, and bow in gratitude.

Zoe found it easy to blame other people—her family, her boss, her friends. But she realized that while others can have an impact, it's really not about anyone else but yourself. "It's about understanding and having compassion for yourself," she says. "I think the compassion thing has come out of having a spiritual practice, learning compassion for myself and other people." Compassion is ultimately a great antidote to anxiety. For women in overdrive, this means compassion for the person they used to be and the person they are becoming, even if they feel they've made "wrong" choices in their lives.

Some women, like Patricia Karnowski, an ovarian cancer survivor, find that trust in their higher self is the key to recovery. After her diagnosis, Patricia would have a nightly "meltdown"—a crying episode that coincided with the setting sun.

"I would just talk to my higher self and say, *Is this really what you want from me?* If this was the right thing, I was okay with it. I did feel like I trusted myself and that there was a connection. I was just in the hands of some bigger force than myself—it wasn't God or Buddha, just a feeling, one that felt secure and safe. I even felt that if I died, it would be okay."

For us overachievers, who often like to have total control of our bodies and environments, this attitude is something that takes time and a major readjustment of a lifetime of patterned thinking. Patricia continues: "My sister died of breast cancer, and my dad died of melanoma. I am okay with that, too. I feel that it's not a bad way to go. People don't wish for cancer. It's kind of a gift. You get a diagnosis, and then you get to live with this urgency about life and love. If I just died, that perspective wouldn't have come to me."

Indeed, for these women, paying attention to their stress levels and illnesses has caused some major changes. Zoe finds she is able to catch herself in the moments when she wants to work to the exclusion of anything else; sometimes she even stops herself. "There is this ironic empowerment that you get when you realize that you can, and must, say no to things. We all know that it's not okay to work 24/7, but we don't really realize the obsessiveness that we practice in our lives. It has no worth, ultimately." Susan says she feels one hundred percent better after leaving her stressful work environment. "I'm sturdier; I feel actually physically stronger. I recognize my limitations and am finally able to say, 'Okay, I have to rest when I have to rest.'"

"Death is our greatest challenge as well as our greatest spiritual opportunity," says Ram Dass, the spiritual leader who wrote the book *Be Here Now.* He wrote these words after suffering from a debilitating stroke that left him wheelchair bound.

As we age, death—or, more appropriately, the prospect of death—leaves us with an entirely new perspective on life. Instead of continuing on a self-destructive trajectory, why not listen to that natural inclination we feel to slow down, spend more time in nature, with family, and pursuing creative interests? This mellowing out allows for introspection, inner growth, and a more positive outcome when it comes to longevity. Learning from those who have been in the trenches, we can come to understand that we don't always have to soldier on. It's like the story of the Tibetan army that, when face to face with the enemy, put flowers in the barrels of their guns and opted for serenity—and good health—instead.

chapter 8:

finding
hormonal
balance

During my pregnancy, strange things have happened to me. Mysterious freckles have appeared on my face. My ligaments have become looser, making me quite bendy in yoga poses that I once found difficult. I often wake up nauseated. I have this strange taste in my mouth that won't go away. I constantly feel thirsty and have an on-again, off-again rash on my abdomen. And those are just the physical symptoms. As for my emotional character, I feel as though possessed by another, less admirable version of myself. I cry if something accidentally falls out of the refrigerator and fly off the handle when my husband doesn't bring me a glass of water *right now*. I have left the front door wide open a few times and recently walked out of a restaurant without paying. But no matter what strange things have happened, every time I call my midwife, she says the same thing: "Oh, that's nothing to worry about. It's totally normal. It's just your hormones."

My husband and I started taking a childbirth class and have learned even more about the role of hormones during pregnancy. A symphony of hormones floods the system at different levels throughout pregnancy and delivery, and after birth. Some help with the pain of childbirth, and others get released during breastfeeding to activate the "mothering response." The amazing world of a woman's hormones made me think about how profound they are at every step of our lives. Of course, the hormonal surges during pregnancy and childbirth are some of the most extreme we'll go through, but what about the rest of our lives? Once we reach puberty, we deal with hormonal fluctuations several times a month. Then come our childbearing years and pregnancy, if we choose to have kids. During perimenopause and menopause comes another series of major hormonal readjustments. Basically, our entire lives we are dealing with major hormonal changes and fluctuations. And when our hormones become out of whack, we suffer from headaches, depression, sleep problems, sexual dysfunction, and moodiness.

It's well established that keeping a hormonal balance is crucial to overall health. Throw in another element of the modern world—high stress—and then what happens? And how do our hormones change over the years, and what we can do to deal with these changes gracefully?

Basically, our entire lives, we

are dealing with major hormonal

changes and fluctuations.

To find the answers to these questions, I spoke at great lengths with Robert A. Greene, MD, a physician specializing in women's issues and the author of *Perfect Balance: Dr. Robert Greene's Breakthrough Program for Finding the Lifelong Hormonal Health You Deserve.*

We started our conversation by talking about life expectancy for women. During the prehistoric period, he told me, the average life expectancy for women was the early teens. During the Iron Age, we lived only into our early twenties. At the time of the Renaissance, we made it until the early thirties. His point in telling me this? We are now living well beyond our natural life expectancy, and that's why our hormones go through so many incredible changes as we age.

Breakdown: Your Hormones

Although they sometimes overlap, here are the four basic hormone groups:

Sex Hormones:
  Estrogen, testosterone, progesterone
Metabolic Hormones:
  Insulin, growth hormone, thyroid hormone
Regulatory Hormones:
  Aldosterone, melatonin, parathyroid hormone
Stress Hormones:
  Cortisol, epinephrine, norepinephrine

Teens Through Thirties

According to Greene, we can trace our hormonal blueprints back to our birth, which begins with a huge surge of estrogen immediately after we are born, lasts a few months, and helps with brain development. Between ages two and nine, sex hormones lie dormant. It's in our teens when things get interesting. "What's happening during the teen years is that everything is being set in motion," explains Greene. "You go through a lot of hormonal chaos in your teen years."

We don't need a doctor to remind us of this fact. If we think hard enough, we can remember the hormonal chaos of adolescence. Outwardly, I became moody, withdrawn, and totally self absorbed. Inwardly, my body began to step up production of follicle-stimulating hormone (FSH) and luteinizing hormone (LH), growth hormone (GH), estrogen, testosterone, and, a few years later, progesterone. All of these together are what bring on the telltale signs of puberty in girls: underarm and pubic hair, breast growth, and our first menstrual cycle.

Greene explains that the reason why these years are so chaotic is that it takes time for the ovaries to establish an adult pattern—and in the meantime, they can respond quite unpredictably. Some months a teen girl has high levels of estrogen; other months they're low; and some months she won't ovulate at all. "The hormone-based communication pattern between the brain and ovaries is maturing, and they are learning to work together," he says.

Once a female reaches her late teens, that dialogue between brain and hormones becomes well rehearsed, and the hormone pattern is predictable. The teens until the late thirties are the major reproductive years, and whether you have kids or not, your hormones will stay relatively consistent. This means that every month, your body prepares for pregnancy as it releases a balance of estrogen, progesterone, and testosterone.

As women approach their late thirties, their fertility rate begins to decline and the hormonal balance isn't as smooth sailing as it used to be. How you feel could depend on how many pregnancies you've had and how many years you've been on the birth control pill. Because ovulation halts when you're pregnant or on the pill, Greene says you don't lose as many eggs, and ultimately your pool of eggs is richer.

The Forties

In our early forties, more changes start to happen in the brain and ovaries. Greene compares this time to the later years of puberty, when you might experience hormonal fluctuations each month—too much estrogen here and too little there—but with one key difference. For a teenager, the frontal lobe of the brain (the area behind your forehead) isn't yet mature; this is the part of the brain that gives us impulse control. "That's why teens may seem so crazy," he says. In our forties, however, this part of the brain has matured. So even though a woman may go through hormonal changes like a teenager, she'll know better than to act on her impulses the second time around.

Although it certainly doesn't happen in only our forties, a word about premenstrual syndrome (PMS) here: Some women have regular menstrual cycles with no symptoms of PMS, while other women get the bloating, breast tenderness, moodiness, and hot flashes associated with it. "The important thing is that the people who have symptoms should know that they are not imagining these problems but instead experiencing a hormonal imbalance," says Greene. "Each person is unique—even identical twins. A lot of what you do—yoga, exercise, food choices—all of these things coalesce into what your individual experience is. Unfortunately, the way medicine has too often dealt with women's issues is to completely marginalize their symptoms." Though some doctors don't treat these problems, others insist that everyone needs a prescription. But each situation varies so dramatically that each woman should determine if her symptoms warrant treatment. This is a very important point, according to Greene, who says that although 80 percent of women in their forties have symptoms of PMS, this doesn't mean that 80 percent need treatment.

According to the survey findings,

1 in 4 Americans turns to food to help

alleviate stress or deal with problems.

In our early to mid-forties, women experience a profound drop in fertility. Although the majority of women continue to have menstrual cycles and the hormone-producing cells in the ovaries are still viable, many are not able to produce a fertile egg.

When women reach this age, estrogen levels actually increase while progesterone levels drop; women also have about half of the testosterone we had at age twenty, according to Greene. As a result, our muscles don't function quite as well and our libido isn't as high. Greene says the drop in testosterone levels is to blame for most of the weight gain and loss of muscle mass. "When testosterone levels are low, we don't need as many calories. But few of us reduce our daily intake to compensate. The net result is, on average, about two pounds per year."

The result of these changes, often overlooked, can be profound—especially for "high-performance" women. "A lot of women, often businesswomen hitting the peaks of their careers, are also dealing with changes in confidence, energy level, and body image," explains Greene. "This is a direct effect of hormonal changes on the brain—estrogen and serotonin levels are more chaotic."

The Fifties

As women get into their late forties, these changes become even more pronounced. Greene tries to avoid the term "menopause," which is technically defined as the twelve-month period after our final menstrual cycle. He doesn't like to use the term because it is really used for research purposes, since you can't define menopause until twelve months *after it has started*. Although it's impossible to tell when a woman will have her last period, science can tell when fertility drops through blood tests that measure hormones. Certain lifestyle factors, such as smoking, can contribute to early menopause. In fact, smokers go into menopause three to five years earlier than nonsmokers. Greene explains that the reason this happens is that tobacco causes the body to convert good estrogen into bad estrogen, essentially turning smokers' own bodies against them.

A woman's fifties are another critical transitional decade when it comes to hormones. This is where the controversial topic of hormone replacement therapy (HRT) comes into play. In 2002, the National Institutes of Health (NIH) discontinued a large, in-progress study examining the effects of a widely used type of HRT medication called Prempro, which combines the hormones estrogen and progestin. The purpose of the study, which was supposed to run until 2005, was to determine whether Prempro would prevent heart disease and hip fractures in women between the ages of fifty and seventy-nine. However, the study was halted because the medicine appeared to increase a woman's risk of breast cancer, heart disease, blood clots, and stroke. Because of the preliminary data showing increased risk of these conditions, the researchers determined that the risks outweighed the benefits. However, this didn't clear things up for most women, since the study recruited women to participate only if they were symptom free so that they could be randomly assigned to take a hormone or a placebo. Today, the consensus is that women taking estrogen and progestin should discuss the condition with their doctors; many believe that the hormone combination is fine for short-term relief of symptoms, since the benefits are likely to outweigh the risks; longer-term use is still in question.[1]

Greene's philosophy is that if you are feeling fine and not having symptoms, you shouldn't be coerced into HRT. "If someone feels good, leave him or her alone," he says. "If they are having symptoms, based on available research, our obligation now is individualizing what we recommend to relieve each person's symptoms, not treating everybody the same."

While one woman may have hot flashes and night sweats, another might suffer from generalized aches and mood changes. Others have a combination. "The important point is that promoting a healthy lifestyle is one of the best ways of reducing the chance of having symptoms," says Greene. "I tell people all of the healthy things they can do. I know a lot of people don't want to make healthy changes—they just want to go to 'quick fix,' so they might jump to hormone therapy more quickly. But the message I promote, the way I can reduce what they need to take and how long they need to take it, is making the healthy changes first."

"One of the simplest things to keep in mind," says Greene, "is that there is literally no hormone that your body makes that can make you feel better at the same time it's harming you! Not the same with drugs. But if a hormone is relieving symptoms and not creating new or different symptoms, then it's not harming your health."

When a woman enters her later fifties, the ovaries aren't producing very many hormones anymore. "Keep in mind that fat cells still produce estrogens, but not the good ones that the brain recognizes. They aren't symptom relieving, and that's why women who are overweight have worse hot flashes," he points out. Greene says another thing that's important to pay attention to is when we need to alter what we do to meet our changing needs. For example, perhaps a woman who hasn't been sexually active gets a new partner, or her long term partner seeks out Viagra. "Then they may need to address symptoms of sexual dysfunction due to inadequate estrogen in order to reduce discomfort from vaginal atrophy. In other words, we may need to change or alter what we recommend to meet each person's changing needs," he says. This doesn't mean that a woman should then seek out hormones as she notices changes that might result from her increase in sexual activity. It's all about relieving symptoms only if they cause distress.

The Sixties and Beyond

As a woman reaches her sixties, her ovaries aren't changing very much. Therefore, any changes in symptoms a woman experiences are related to external factors, for example, stress levels, dietary patterns, or loss of a partner. As we age, many women also develop disturbances associated with thyroid dysfunction or rising insulin levels. Each person's hormonal changes also reflect individual genetic risks, as well as the long-term effects of bad habits. For instance, many women experience rising blood pressure problems due to hormones like angiotensin, which is made by the liver. To further complicate aging, each hormonal shift may trigger changes in other hormones, creating further hormone chaos. The good news is that if we pay attention to symptoms, specific interventions can restore balance and promote healthy aging and longevity.

A Little Knowledge

All of these hormonal changes in a woman's life mean we are constantly dealing with their physical and emotional results. Whether you are a teen going through puberty or a sixty-year-old trying to wean yourself off HRT, it's easy to see how our hormones play a major role in how we feel and operate in the world.

I'm the kind of person who needs an explanation for everything. If I feel out of sorts, I try to trace it back to my actions: Did I eat too much? Sleep poorly? Forget to drink my morning tea? For me, learning about the impact of hormones on a woman's health felt like somewhat of a relief. I suspect that I'm not the only one. With so many changes going on daily, monthly, yearly, and through the decades, it's no wonder we women have such vastly differing experiences from one day to the next. And our hormones don't just stop changing once we leave the front door. They affect everything we do—at work, with our families, with our children. Not that we have a "get-out-of-jail-free card" for acting irrationally, but the awareness that these fluctuations are happening can help us to remove the veil of self-criticism so many of us fall prey to.

Whether you are a teen going through puberty or a 60-year-old trying to wean yourself off HRT, it's easy to see how our hormones play a major role in how we feel and operate in the world.

The key is self-acceptance: Instead of

fearing the changes or trying to deny them,

we can try to go with the flow and discover

what makes us feel good, happy, and whole,

instead of focusing on what makes us

feel inadequate and out of control.

Poses for Reduced Anxiety

1. STANDING FORWARD BEND

Stand in Mountain Pose with your hands on your hips. Exhale and bend forward from the hip joints. Emphasize lengthening the front torso as you move more fully into the position. Bring the fingertips to the floor slightly in front of you or cross your forearms and hold your elbows. Press the heels firmly into the floor and lift the sitting bones toward the ceiling. Let your head hang from the root of the neck, which is deep in the upper back, between the shoulder blades. With each inhalation lift and lengthen the front torso slightly; with each exhalation release a little more fully into the forward bend. Stay for thirty seconds to one minute.

2. SUPPORTED BRIDGE POSE

You'll need two bolsters and two blankets. To set up, place the bolsters end to end to accommodate the length of your body. Depending on your flexibility, you can increase the backbend by adding bolsters or blankets on top. Sit down, straddling the bolsters, and move slightly nearer

to the end behind you. Use the support of your arms to help you lie down. Carefully slide off the end toward your head so your shoulders touch the floor and you face the ceiling. Don't jam your chin into your chest; you can use a rolled-up towel under the base of your neck for support. Place an eye bag over your eyes. Let your eyeballs turn downward. Bring your attention to the breath; feel the lateral movement of your lungs and ribs with each breath. Stay here for fifteen minutes.

3. CORPSE POSE WITH RAISED LEGS

Lie on your back facing a chair or couch. Lift your legs, and prop your calves up on the chair or couch. To support your neck, put a rolled-up towel at the base of your neck, parallel to your shoulders. Cover your eyes with an eye bag. If you have tension in your lower back, place a blanket under the backs of the knees. Bring your arms out to the sides, palms facing up. Relax your jaw, soften your eyelids, and release the root of your tongue. Allow the legs to roll outward. Take deep breaths and allow yourself to melt into the floor. Stay here for 15 - 20 minutes.

The weight gain of pregnancy that's hard to lose, the loss of self-confidence in the workplace during our forties, or the negative feelings of aging during menopause are often due to hormones. Even if we are used to feeling great, our hormones can make us feel out of control and a bit batty. The key is self-acceptance: Instead of fearing the changes or trying to deny them, we can try to go with the flow and discover what makes us feel good, happy, and whole instead of focusing on what makes us feel inadequate and out of control.

Stress Hormones and Women's Health

Beyond the many facets of female hormones throughout our lives, we also have another type of hormones coursing through our bodies. "One of the most important things people should realize is that stress is a hormonal condition," says Greene. When we perceive danger, our brain floods our body with the stress hormones epinephrine, norepinephrine, and cortisol. These hormones trigger changes in heart rate, blood patterns, and digestive patterns. The result is feeling "stressed out," tired, irritable, and possibly out of control.

Of course, how we manifest stress is different in every person. Some of us get headaches and ulcers; others get panic attacks and upset stomachs. The "stress response," which causes stress to elevate, is a reflex that has helped us survive over the centuries and is still called the "fight-or-flight response." We've all heard the story about how this response occurred during evolution: When we needed to respond quickly to danger that

Natural Remedies for Stress

Need to calm down *now*? Try the following natural solutions for stressful situations:

Rescue Remedy: Take a few drops of this flower essence when experiencing anxiety before or after a stressful event to calm your nerves (www .bach.com).

Herbs: Valerian, chamomile, skullcap, Saint John's wort, passionflower. Buy these herbs and boil them for tea; they also can be bought in tinctures or capsules at your local health-food store.

Packaged Tea: If you don't want the hassle of making your own tea, try some teas that contain calming ingredients. I like Yogi Tea's Bedtime Tea (www .yogitea.com), which has valerian and skullcap. St. John's Good Mood by Traditional Medicinals (www.traditionalmedicinals.com) has Saint John's wort, lemon balm, and English lavender, which help with nervousness. Another favorite is Tension Tamer by Celestial Seasonings (www .celestialseasonings.com), which has lots of B vitamins and calming herbs.

threatened our survival, such as a lion chasing after us, our stress hormones kicked into high gear so we wouldn't die. This response evolved so the species would survive.

But today, though we have different "lions"—traffic, work, a high-stakes meeting, a fight with a telemarketer, issues with a stepchild, high mortgage payments, mothers-in-law—they cause the same flooding of stress hormones. And what's worse, instead of dealing with the issue of an oncoming lion maybe once or twice a year, some of us feel the stress response many times a day. Thus, our stress response is unnaturally high, leading to all sorts of conditions that threaten our overall well-being and lead to all sorts of stress-related conditions. When the fight-or-flight response is used inappropriately, however, it can lead to some devastating conditions.[2] Greene explains it this way: "When stress hormones are *briefly* elevated, they promote memory formation, motivation, and energy production. When they are *chronically* elevated, on the other hand—a situation that's increasingly common in our fast-paced, multitasking world—they can become toxic and adversely affect our emotional state, memory, and even sleep patterns."

How to counter the stress response? Trigger the Relaxation Response, a technique akin to meditation that Dr. Herbert Benson popularized in the seventies and that was fashioned after Transcendental Meditation.

Although it's been around a while, Benson's *The Relaxation Response* is still one of the most important and oft-cited books around when it comes to stress. The result of the Relaxation Response—essentially, focusing the mind on a phrase or sound for ten to twenty minutes—includes physiological effects like slowed heartbeat and breathing, reduced oxygen consumption, and increased skin resistance. But beyond these physical effects, the Relaxation Response leaves us feeling soothed. And this isn't a new phenomenon. According to Benson's book, this state has been routinely experienced in both Eastern and Western cultures throughout time, and people who've experienced it have reported ecstasy, clairvoyance, and total relaxation.

Yoga for Lowering Stress Hormones

Chronic anxiety can wreak havoc on our physical, emotional, and spiritual well-being. One way to reduce the chronic anxiety that contributes to heightened stress hormones is a practice like yoga. Of course, women with serious anxiety should be under the care of a physician, but yoga is a perfect fit for those of us with that constant underlying harried feeling. "The overarching principle is this," says Judith Lasater, PhD, yoga teacher, physical therapist, and author of many books on yoga, including *Relax and Renew: Restful Yoga for Stressful Times*: "It is physiologically impossible to be anxious and relaxed at the same time. They are polar opposites. In the short term, relaxation reduces anxiety, but it offers long-term benefits as well. When you regularly practice relaxation, you create a habit of paying attention to your inner state. Thus you notice more quickly that you are becoming anxious and tense, and you can take steps to alleviate this."

As we know, anxiety activates the sympathetic nervous system and our bodies are flooded with stress hormones to prepare the body for the fight-or-flight response. Yoga practices can counteract this reaction by stimulating the parasympathetic nervous system, which elicits the Relaxation Response. Yoga also helps alleviate anxiety because we hold tension in our muscles: When we stretch the muscles, combined with long, slow breathing, the muscles—and therefore tension—release.

Yoga helps to ground an overactive and anxious mind by giving it something to focus on. But Lasater warns against overdoing it in an attempt to lessen anxiety. "People believe that if they are still it will just make them feel their pain more. They try to 'burn it off' with vigorous exercise, mistaking exhaustion for relaxation. But this strategy only works short term, and they may still experience sleep and digestive ramifications, as well as other symptoms of stress," she says. Inversions and other restorative yoga poses, which lower the head below the heart, are usually experienced as relaxing. Forward bends also bring the mind inward and help you to shut out the rest of the world and the worries that go along with it. "When you are anxious your thoughts are directed toward the future and are about what might happen," says Lasater. "We need to practice learning to go inside and focus on the here and now, which is not a skill taught in our culture." Chest openers like backbends help to open the diaphragm and facilitate deep breathing, which can lead to a calmer nervous system. "According to traditional yoga wisdom, whatever is low is quieted, so lower your head to slow your brain," adds Lasater. Whatever pose you choose, always pay close attention to the breath. And avoid Inversions during pregnancy and menstruation.

Your Stress Hormones

1. **Cortisol** is a hormone produced by the adrenal glands, located just above the kidneys. It aids in metabolism, maintains blood pressure, and helps to manage stress——when you feel stressed, cortisol levels in the body increase.

2. **Epinephrine**, the hormone also known as adrenaline, is released into the bloodstream by the adrenal gland during the fight-or-flight response. It allows the body to get ready to fight or run during a threat: The heart starts to pump harder, blood pressure increases, airways in the lungs open, blood vessels narrow, and blood flows to major muscle groups.

3. **Norepinephrine**, both a hormone and a neuro-transmitter, is also known as noradrenaline. It's secreted by the adrenal medulla into the blood-stream as part of the fight-or-flight response.

Regulating Your Hormones

Reacting to the stress hormones surging through our bodies takes awareness and consciousness. Practices like yoga, breathing, and tai chi dramatically lower stress hormones and positively affect the immune, cardiovascular, and digestive systems, allowing the body to get out of "danger mode" and back into its normal pattern. Greene points to exercise as crucial in keeping the hormones balanced. "It's important to start from a point of biological plausibility. We are all basically descendants of hunter-gatherers—there is no idleness there. During the average day, people were traveling great distances and doing physical work." Today, says Greene, we spend all day moving from one *chair* to another! Over the years, he points out, our physiology hasn't changed, but our diet and way of life have. With a high-calorie diet and sedentary lifestyle, we have strayed from our evolutionary roots.

We are beginning to understand the details about how exercise affects our hormonal balance; neither too much nor too little, but rather a balanced approach is best. Greene looks at the changing landscape of research in this area; he says that fifteen years ago the official recommendation for pregnant women was to walk thirty minutes twice a week! Today, this has been modified to at least forty-five minutes every day. Since Benson's book was published in 1975, a huge amount of research on stress hormones and these practices has been conducted to prove how relaxation practices can lower stress hormones.

Studies on Stress

Hundreds of studies on the effects of stress have been done. Here are a few interesting ones:

Psychologist Salvatore R. Maddi, PhD, showed that "hardiness" is the key to thriving under stress. In a twelve-year study that followed downsized employees from Illinois Bell Telephone, results showed that about two-thirds of the employees in the study suffered significant performance, leadership, and health declines as the result of the extreme stress from downsizing, including heart attacks, strokes, obesity, depression, substance abuse, and poor performance reviews. However, the other one-third actually thrived during the same upheaval, maintaining their health, happiness, and performance; they even reportedly felt renewed enthusiasm. Maddi found three key beliefs among those who thrived and turned adversity into advantage: They stayed involved in ongoing events, rather than isolating themselves; they tried to influence and control outcomes, rather than lapsing into passivity and powerlessness; and they viewed stress changes, whether positive or negative, as opportunities for new learning.[3]

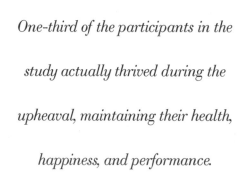

One-third of the participants in the

study actually thrived during the

upheaval, maintaining their health,

happiness, and performance.

A national survey by the American Psychological Association in partnership with the National Women's Health Resource Center and iVillage.com showed that people dealt with stress by engaging in unhealthy behaviors such as comfort eating, poor diet choices, smoking, and inactivity. And those who experienced stress were more likely to report hypertension, anxiety or depression, and obesity. Among the most interesting findings? Women reported feeling the effects of stress on their physical health more than men. One in four Americans turns to food to help alleviate stress or deal with problems; comfort eaters report higher levels of stress than average and exhibit higher levels of all the most common symptoms of stress, including fatigue, lack of energy, nervousness, irritability, and trouble sleeping. Forty-seven percent of Americans say they are concerned about stress. Fifty-one percent of women say stress affects them, compared to 43 percent of men. Women dealing with stress report feelings of nervousness, a desire to cry, or lack of energy, while men talk about having trouble sleeping or feeling irritable or angry. And women are more likely than men to report health problems related to stress, such as hypertension, anxiety or depression, and obesity.[4]

A recent study by neuroscientists at Harvard Medical School and McLean Hospital has shown that long-term exposure to stress hormones in mice directly results in the anxiety that often comes with depression.[5]

The list of negative effects of stress goes on. Stress has been linked to heart attacks, depression, diminished immunity, and increased cholesterol. But we don't need a study to tell us that too much stress makes us feel bad. And we know that thinking positively and nurturing ourselves make us feel better. On the following pages are a few more ways we can lower our stress hormones on a day-to-day basis.

Ten Stress-Busters

1. Don't multitask. When you find yourself doing more than one thing at a time——like talking on the phone and driving, or cooking dinner and watching television——stop. Ask yourself which activity is more important, and focus on that one.

2. Clean out your space. Often a messy desk or a crammed closet contributes to feelings of lack of control, frustration, and plain old stress. Clear out your space to clear out your mind.

3. Sit up straight. Often slumping can lead to shallow breathing. This often means headaches, backaches, and unnecessary stress. When you have good posture, you can breathe deeply throughout the day——a guaranteed way to feel more relaxed.

4. Start the day right. Instead of jumping straight out of bed, choose one thing that feels good: Stretch in bed, taking three deep breaths; make a cup of tea and sit in the back yard; snuggle with your kitty. Whatever you choose, it doesn't have to take long, but starting out slowly and mindfully can change the tenor of your entire day.

5. Practice random acts of kindness. In life's hustle-bustle, we often forget how good it feels to give. For one day, smile at strangers. Leave an extra-big tip at the coffee shop. Write a friend an email telling her how much you appreciate her.

6. Listen to music. Music has the power to transform a mood. Turn on your favorite relaxing music and watch the stress melt away.

7. Stay positive. When you see the glass as half full instead of half empty, you're likely to feel less stress and more excitement about life.

8. Express yourself. Instead of suppressing your emotions like anger and sadness, set them free. Talk to a friend or therapist; you might be surprised at how good it feels.

9. Take a bath. Rejoice in the water while you listen to music or read your favorite magazine.

10. Laugh. Remember how good it felt as a kid to laugh many times a day? Try to recapture this playful spirit.

chapter 9

hop off
the
treadmill

As I finish writing this book, I am now the proud and somewhat awestruck mother of a newborn son named Lucian. And
my understanding and awareness of overdrive have taken on
a whole new dimension as I try to combine new motherhood
and fluctuating hormones with the more familiar routines of
housework, marriage, and deadlines. Hopping off the treadmill
seems like a distant goal, one that even as I attended childbirth
preparation classes I was aware would be a challenge for me
and the women around me.

I remember how, during my weekly childbirth preparation
class, the moms-to-be went around the room to talk about how
we were feeling during our pregnancies. We talked about how
our backs hurt, our emotions were haywire, we couldn't sleep
well, and we had to pee every half hour. We all struggled for
ways to deal with the physical and emotional changes while
holding down jobs, spending time with our partners, taking
care of other children, and maintaining friendships. Women in
overdrive all of us were—it was obvious—and we couldn't or
wouldn't give anything up. Often we can't because of financial concerns or obligations we can't simply drop. And often
we won't because we want it all—a great career, a wonderful

marriage, a rewarding job, a close-knit family. And we deserve these things. But we also have to be careful. One woman in the group stands out in my mind. An architect, she takes the bus to work and works at a drawing table where she stands on her feet all day every day. That day in class, close to her due date, she told the group: "Even though I feel so huge and it's hard to walk and my back hurts, this is the first time in my life I've slowed down." She went on to tell us that she secretly wishes the baby will arrive late, just so she can enjoy some more time to herself.

This is a radical example, but doing something for ourselves, where we can take time off and reset our clocks, often happens only at major transitional times like pregnancy. But as women in overdrive, we may approach our relaxation with the same sense of overachievement we bring to other areas of our lives. Last week, after a grueling week of working, taking care of my infant, and generally keeping my household, relationships, and work life functioning, I decided to escape to a local Japanese bathhouse for its weekly women-only day. But when I got there, I confronted a long waiting list. It seemed that I wasn't the only one looking for relaxation. Dozens of women sat around, eagerly waiting for their name to be called so they could get their chance at slowing down. Women in overdrive seek out these experiences—yoga retreats, meditation weekends, trips to the local bathhouse—with an urgent desperation. We feel as if we need to escape our circumstances and *then* we can relax. When constantly running on overdrive, we often approach our "downtime" with the same drive and determination. But what would it be like if we could incorporate a feeling of balance and relaxation into our everyday lives?

Women in overdrive tend to keep moving forward. But I would love to see us consciously choose to stop the cycle. In our hectic lives, a major break to restore ourselves through giving ourselves a quick emotional cleansing doesn't just happen. Finding balance in this burnout culture requires some planning, ingenuity, and commitment.

Finding balance in this

burnout culture requires some planning,

ingenuity, and commitment.

Emotional Cleansing

When we think of a cleansing, we often think in terms of our physical bodies—perhaps a juice fast to clear out the digestive system, or a week of back-to-back yoga classes to wring out accumulated toxins. But before we work on our bodies, experts say, it's important to focus on our emotions. "The physical and mental levels will take care of themselves most of the time," Richard Faulds, a senior teacher at Kripalu Center for Yoga & Health and the author of *Kripalu Yoga: A Guide to Practice On and Off the Mat,* told me. "If we do the emotional work, the other levels tend to blossom."

Whether it's weight, work, or relationship issues, we all have our burdens to bear. But for many of us there comes a point when these burdens start to interfere, preventing us from experiencing the full range of life's richness. "Carrying around unresolved issues from the past makes life less enjoyable," says David Simon, cofounder and medical director of the Chopra Center for Wellbeing at the La Costa Resort & Spa in Carlsbad, California, and leader of a workshop called "Healing the Heart." "If you are always nursing these issues, it becomes impossible to become completely open and available to what's happening in your present," he adds.

And when we find ourselves so stuck on the past that we can't enjoy the present, an emotional cleansing may be the key to helping us move forward.

Out with the Old, In with the New

According to Simon, emotional toxicity comes from feeling our needs aren't being met. "A history of accumulated unmet needs erodes your sense of vitality, self-esteem, and sense of worthiness," says Simon, "and this creates some emotional residue." It may seem that a little emotional residue isn't such a bad thing, but carrying it around can cause us to build up so much armor that we miss out on a huge range of experiences. "When you have emotional blocks that prevent you from inhabiting your full range of emotions, you lose the low notes—but you also lose the high notes," says Faulds. "If you lose the ability to feel sadness, you lose the ability to feel bliss."

Faulds compares holding on to toxic emotions to dragging a beach ball deeper and deeper under water, which increases pressure on the ball. "When emotion is blocked, the pressure gets higher and higher and tends to aggravate the mind, and we walk around with an emotional charge. This pressurizes your psyche and makes you more reactive."

Flying off the handle isn't the only result of chronic emotional toxicity; storing these emotions can have devastating physical effects. At Kripalu, Faulds sees visitors with unresolved emotional baggage suffering from all sorts of ailments, including chronic neck and back pain, migraine headaches, chronic fatigue, insomnia, low immune response, anxiety attacks, panic attacks, and depression.

"When you have emotional blocks

that prevent you from inhabiting your

full range of emotions, you lose the low

notes—but you also lose the high notes,"

says Faulds. "If you lose the ability to feel

sadness, you lose the ability to feel bliss."

Cleansing 101

Many options exist when it comes to getting rid of emotional baggage. But some say that putting aside a concentrated period of time works better than anything else they've tried in the past. "You can be in therapy for years and read all of the self-help books you want, and you still can't get there," says Evelyn Kelly, a forty-one-year-old actress living in Los Angeles who also attended Simon's workshop. Of course, undoing the process of years of building up toxic emotions doesn't happen in a weekend, but here are a few ideas to help facilitate the process:

Choose to address your issues.

It would be easy to go through life brushing our emotional issues under the table—and many of us do. But sometimes we reach a turning point where we must move forward. "Usually it reaches a point where the pain of ignoring it outweighs the pain of dealing with it," says Simon. This point sometimes comes after a specific event, such as a divorce, the death of a loved one, or job loss. For others, the decision comes when we've simply had enough. Still others have an inkling that something is missing from their lives. "Some people have a feeling there is more out there and make a decision to live differently," says Faulds.

Create a safe environment.

Once you are ready to confront your emotions, the next step is to foster a supportive place. "If you create an environment that's very safe, your defense mechanisms can relax and start to heal," says Simon. A safe space could involve a trip to a place like the Chopra Center or Kripalu Center for Yoga & Health, where a trained staff, along with the company of others on the same path, creates a loving atmosphere. If getting away isn't possible, create a space at home by setting aside a weekend where you clear your schedule and unplug your phone—whatever helps you disengage from your active and demanding life.

Identify your toxins.

Once you are in an environment that will support your cleansing, take part in activities that will help you identify your issues. Choose not to read the paper, watch television, or engage in conversations that will sap your energy. Instead, use that time to write in a journal, listen to soothing music, eat healthy foods, get a massage, and do some yoga or deep breathing. "These things can create the space you need to identify your issues and bring into more conscious awareness both the feelings and the patterns tied to a perpetual sense of emotional stress and lack of fulfillment," says Simon.

Meditate.

Experts agree that meditation is a key to quieting down the inner turbulence that gets in the way of living life to the fullest. "Ask questions to listen to the deep inner voice for responses, hear something from inside that surprised you," says Simon. He says sometimes during meditation a memory suddenly bursts into awareness, giving a student insight into his or her past or the answer to a question that has been lingering. "That kind of experience gives people the confidence that old patterns don't have to continue."

Be honest.

The process of clearing out toxins requires brutal honesty. After quieting down, Kelly discovered the root of her emotional baggage. She was one of seven children, and her mother became sick when Kelly was six, with an illness that lasted for the next twelve years. As a result, Kelly never felt that she got enough attention. "Because of that, I started to internalize things, like *I must not be good enough; otherwise I would get more of my mother's attention,*" she says. After she was honest with herself about the root of her feelings of insecurity, she was able to see how this scenario played itself out in her adult relationships. "I now realize that we all are worthy of the kind of love that we deserve."

Release.

Once you've identified the toxicity, create a ritual to release it. This could mean throwing rocks in the ocean, writing a letter and burning it, calling somebody you've been avoiding— anything that will help you consciously let go and symbolize that things are shifting. "We can access and express through ritual things that are oftentimes too challenging, too threatening otherwise," says Faulds. "It's a way to powerfully express emotion and action."

Commit to new choices.

Once you've released your toxins, it's important to commit yourself to not re-creating them. "It's great to have insight and feel some relief, but the long-term benefits of the healing process are clearly about making a commitment. It's too easy to have a relapse," says Simon, whose book *The Ten Commitments: Translating Good Intentions into Great Choices* covers this topic. To do this, create an intention to honor your commitment and develop discipline to stick to it.

A cleansing will leave you feeling rejuvenated and more alive. "The energy that was being used to suppress the pain is now available for creative options," says Simon, who has witnessed his students make radical changes in their relationships, work, and health as a result of an emotional cleansing.

Physical Cleansing

Recently, I saw Mireille Guiliano, the author of *French Women Don't Get Fat: The Secret of Eating for Pleasure,* on a talk show. She answers the question millions of American women have: How do French women, whose diet consists of croissants, brie, and red wine, stay so slim? Her answer: French women treat food as pleasurable instead of guilt inducing. According to her, French women walk a lot, balance out one heavy meal with a lighter one, and instead of weighing themselves just depend on how their clothing fits. I had to laugh at the common sense of it all. Deprivation leads to overindulgence, and most American women I know struggle with issues of guilt and self-hatred around food. I don't think I'm stating this too strongly. Skinny or fat, it seems that we start from a young age to have a love/hate relationship with food. I can remember events in my life based on my weight: I was thin in high school, heavy in college, thin again in grad school, even thinner when I moved to California, and now, well, after the pregnancy we'll see how it goes. The point is that this tenuous relationship wastes so much energy: Eat a piece of cake and then feel guilty. Don't eat it and feel virtuous.

It's not hard to overeat. When we go to a restaurant, the portions are huge. We eat at buffets and takeout restaurants. Most women in overdrive would probably say we care about nutrition but lack the time to nourish ourselves properly. I often eat in front of the computer or eat things I really don't want, like a bagel or a pastry, just because it's in front of me—and it's fast.

When food becomes a means of compulsion and addiction, the cycle never seems to end. When I eat a lot of sugar or carbohydrates, I want more. When I eat something I've labeled as "bad" for me, I feel guilty and like a failure. I often eat mindlessly while on the phone, or keep making short trips to the refrigerator when I'm working in order to procrastinate.

As a woman in overdrive, I have also noticed that I sometimes treat food as a reward: A finished article, a busy day completed, a celebration—all seem like good reasons to overindulge.

Over the years, I've found that a fast can reset my clock when it comes to food. It can clear out toxins, cleanse the blood, and restore vitality to many organs of the body. For some of us, the idea of a fast seems too radical. I have tried fasts where I didn't eat for a day or period of days, but these didn't work for me. Now the fasts I choose always include some amounts of food rather than total abstinence. Carrie L'Esperance, in her book *The Ancient Cookfire,* includes the following quote by George Ottawa, which expresses what a fast means to me: "Real fasting does not entail giving up eating and drinking entirely. Fasting means abandonment of the habit of greed, which causes us always to eat and drink in excess; fasting in the true sense means to eat and drink simply in accord with those principles, which are at the core of the infinite order of the universe. Fasting, too, is an antidote to overeating."

Toxins accumulate in our bodies as the result of stress, the environment, overeating, and drugs and alcohol. When we become toxic, our systems are adversely affected because oxidation doesn't happen in the tissues, leaving us tired and fatigued. Restoring the body through a fast can help to reverse these effects. "The principle of fasting is based on the basic structures and processes of the human body, mind, and spirit," writes L'Esperance. "Some people confuse fasting with starvation and find various ways to talk themselves out of this healthful practice. The sense of hunger often disappears in people who completely abstain from food—both those fasting and those starting—but the similarity ends there. The process of fasting is one of gradually aligning more and more with the body. It is actually the epitome of a natural way of life, and its benefits do not end by correcting our out-of-balance systems and restoring our health."[1]

I have done dozens of fasts over my lifetime, and they are difficult because they require restraint and discipline. But I look at fasts as a time to slow down and take it easy. You really have no choice—when eating less food than normal, you feel a bit sluggish and low on energy. I love the mental picture of my body as a series of pipes: A fast gets rid of what's clogging and congesting my system, clearing the way so that my body feels pure and clean.

In the beginning, I started fasting for one day once a week. When my schedule wouldn't allow this anymore, I fasted about once a month over the weekend. I did the same fast: no food, only water and broth. But soon I learned that fasting can coincide with the seasons, and that each season corresponds with a certain organ or organs. After I fast, my body automatically seems to reset. I crave less sugar, refined foods, and animal fats. I find that simple whole grains and vegetables fill me up and leave me feeling satisfied.

Seasonal Fasts

Here are examples of seasonal fasts for spring and fall, based on the helpful book by Carrie L'Esperance, who told me that these seasons are the most powerful times to cleanse the body When you fast, remember that it's a special time to relax and renew. Try to cut down, or eliminate, if possible, as much activity as you can. Write in a journal, go for long walks, meditate, and envision your body being cleaned out.

According to the Chinese five-element theory, each season corresponds to different organs, and these fasts are based on the idea that they should be cleansed during the appropriate season. Try to get fresh, organic fruits and vegetables when you use them.

Spring Equinox Fast

Organ: Gall bladder and liver

Time Frame: One to three days

8 AM to noon: Kiwis, oranges, limes, grapefruit, lemons, apples, pure water, and herbal teas. Take these in either solid or liquid form. Eat and drink as much as you like until noon.

Noon to 8 PM: Asparagus, beets, broccoli, cabbage, cauliflower, dandelion leaves, garlic, olive oil, parsley, sprouts, pure water, and herbal teas. The vegetables can be raw, steamed, baked, or roasted, and a dressing can be made from olive oil, garlic, and parsley. It is best to have a combination of raw and cooked foods at each meal to supply the live enzymes needed for proper digestion.

Menu to break the fast: Add spring grains like barley, quinoa, wheat, millet, and rye. Eat plain yogurt flavored with vanilla extract and spices, goat's milk cheeses, and free-range chicken, turkey, or fish.

Autumn Fast

Organs: Lungs, large intestine

Time frame: Three days

According to L'Esperance, pineapple and pineapple juice are good for lung problems, high blood pressure, and tumors.

Eat as much fresh pineapple as you want. Supplement this with wormwood and ginger tea, figs, raw almonds, and whole pumpkin seeds. Take a strong laxative tea or frozen castor oil capsules the morning or night of the third day, and the rest of the days following if you choose to continue this fast for a longer period of time.

Menu to break the fast: Add spring grains like barley, quinoa, wheat, millet, and rye. Eat plain yogurt flavored with vanilla extract and spices, goat's milk cheeses, and free-range chicken or turkey.

L'Esperance believes that fruits, vegetables, and herbs are the most cleansing foods we have. Unlike meats, dairy, and fats, they don't take a lot of energy to digest and get absorbed into the bloodstream quickly. If you really want to do a simple cleansing and you don't have a lot of time, try doing this mini-fast: Eat only fruits, or only vegetables, or drink only herbal tea for one day. Or, she says, you can mix up these three ingredients throughout the day. For example, a one-day fast might mean eating only fruit in the morning and vegetables in the afternoon and drinking herbal teas with detoxifying properties, such as sarsaparilla, all day long. Make sure the tea is medicinal strength—three tablespoons of herbs per two cups of water. These herbs are stronger than vitamins and difficult to integrate into your diet (did you ever hear of a recipe that calls for sarsaparilla?), so teas are a great way to get them into your diet.

Stress and Your Diet

"When you have stress, your body needs ten times more nutrition than when you don't have stress," L'Esperance told me. For women in overdrive, this means getting enough of the "stress" vitamins, C, E, and B. But this still isn't enough; if you don't have enough minerals in your body, you can't absorb the vitamins. Of course, you can always take a capsule. But it's also a good idea to obtain these vitamins and minerals from your diet because they are absorbed more easily into the body. To do this, branch out into foods you might not have yet in your cupboard: wheat germ, brewer's yeast, fresh walnuts, organic raisins, medicinal teas, and whole grains.

Women in overdrive should also eat a diet high in protein that includes beans, tofu, fresh fish, and lean chicken—preferably organic to avoid antibiotics. "The carbs are where people get into trouble," L'Esperance told me. The ubiquity of breads, cakes, white rice, potatoes, and sweets presents a major challenge to most mere mortals.

"It's difficult to stay in balance when everything else around you is out of balance," she acknowledges.

As we know, women in overdrive tend to overdo it. A fast shouldn't be an impossible task; it should be done lovingly, within the confines of your health and well-being. Your fast must be suited to your body and the time in your life. If you choose it, you won't be disappointed. "If you are reasonably well, most fasts will bring about an almost euphoric feeling of well-being and provide inexpensive and effective insurance against disease," says L'Esperance. "If you are not well, the fast is an excellent beginning of a therapeutic program."

And just because your fast is over doesn't mean you should go back to binge eating. "The big mistake that people make is that they don't have a varied diet," says L'Esperance. So continue eating lots of fruits and veggies, yummy teas, and protein sources in lots of combinations so you don't get bored, and eat seasonal foods to stay in touch with nature. Drop the idea that fat is "bad"! We need fats in our diet, so incorporate "good" oils, like hemp seed, flax, sesame, or pumpkin.

Perhaps even more important for women in overdrive is finding the time to prepare healthy meals at home. "Once you stop cooking for yourself, it's really hard to stay in balance," says L'Esperance. When we go out, we gravitate toward prepared food we might never eat at home—that bagel in the coffee shop with colleagues or a steak out to dinner with friends. When you cook at home, you know exactly what you are putting into your body.

Eating as You Age

As we get older, it's a good idea to eat four or five smaller meals a day, rather than two or three big ones. L'Esperance told me that as we age, our digestion diminishes, which is exacerbated by a pattern of not eating right throughout our lives. "The body reaches its physical peak at twenty-one, and then everything begins to diminish and slow down—unless you do prevention."

She recommends taking digestive enzymes with papaya, pineapple, and peppermint after meals to aid in digestion. And when it comes to getting protein, avoid heavy meats and gravitate toward fish, egg yolks, sheep's milk, and cheeses. Also, stay away from artificial sweeteners that many women consume because they think they will help them stay slim as they age. "Women are destroying themselves," says L'Esperance. "Artificial sweeteners penetrate the blood/brain barrier and destroy the immune system." She believes as well that cell phones, computers, and antennas all serve to break down the body as we age.

Kitchari

The kitchari fast has been my favorite one over the years. This delicious and hearty soup is a combination of rice, mung beans, and spices that has been used for centuries to purify digestion, clean out toxins, and restore balance to the body. It works because you can still get the proper nourishment while allowing your body to heal. Kitchari, like any mono-fast where you eat only one thing, gives the body a rest from processing different foods.

RECIPE:

1. Rinse and soak one cup of split yellow mung beans for several hours. Set aside.

2. Liquefy one tablespoon of peeled, chopped ginger; two tablespoons of shredded coconut; and a handful of chopped cilantro with one-half cup of water in a blender.

She also reminds us that part of how we age is determined by genetics. So look at your family's history: Is there heart disease? Diabetes? Use this information not to worry about, but to tailor, your diet and lifestyle.

Ultimately, whether you are a woman in overdrive or not, eating a healthful diet is a constant struggle. "You have a baby

3. In a large saucepan, lightly brown one-half
   teaspoon cinnamon; one-quarter teaspoon each
   of cardamom, pepper, clove powder, turmeric,
   and salt; and three bay leaves (remove before
   serving) in three tablespoons of ghee, or
   butter.

4. Drain the beans and then stir them into the
   spice mixture in the saucepan.

5. Add one cup of raw basmati rice.

6. Stir in the blended spice and coconut mixture,
   followed by six cups of water.

7. Bring to a boil, cover, and cook on low heat for
   approximately 25 to 30 minutes until soft.

and that throws you off," says L'Esperance. "Your partner has a situation and that throws you off. It's a constant challenge to stay in balance, and so the best thing that people can do is be careful about what decisions they make in their lives." What she is really saying is not to bite off more than you can chew so that you live in a constant state of being overwhelmed.

Foods for Adrenal Glands

Our adrenal glands are often depleted because we operate so much of the time in fight-or-flight response. If you feel tired or exhausted often, your adrenals might be to blame. Try eating the following foods, rich in panothenic acid, to feed your adrenals: beets, spinach, celery, carrots, mushrooms, split peas, soybeans, broccoli, kale, and cauliflower. These vitamin C-rich foods also help with stress: peppers, parsley, brussels sprouts, citrus fruits, and strawberries.

Eating with Awareness

If you don't have time to fast, you can still eat with awareness to nourish your spirit and transform your life. Every single mealtime provides us with the opportunity for waking up in smaller but no less important ways. "Mindfulness while eating can become a truly transformational practice," says Halé Sofia Schatz, nourishment educator and author of *If the Buddha Came to Dinner,* "because we can then align our mind, heart, and physical body—and from that place we can nourish and revitalize ourselves at a deep level."

The body reaches its physical

peak at 21, and then everything

begins to diminish and slow

down—unless you do prevention.

Coming to this deep place of alignment takes more than just the standard advice to chew slowly a hundred times before swallowing. "It really has very little to do with the actual foods," Schatz explained to me. "It's more of a relationship with ourselves." So how do we establish this kind of relationship to get the nourishment we crave? To start, we can reduce the amount of foods we eat that pollute the environment, such as meat—raising cattle causes water pollution, erosion, and deforestation and genetically modified foods, which are destroying many indigenous variations of seeds. We can also choose foods like organic fruits or free range chicken that don't pollute our bodies with pesticides or synthetic growth hormones. We can simplify mealtimes by eating less at each sitting, limiting the choice of foods we consume, and not going back for seconds. When it comes to eating, we can employ the same kind of discipline we use to keep our jobs, raise our families, and learn an instrument. Because all new skills require a measure of discipline, we can treat mindful eating as something new we are practicing for the long-term goal of finding freedom from cravings, overeating, and obsessive thoughts about food. "To feed ourselves in a way that respects our inherent need for balance, we have to set limits for ourselves," says Schatz, who calls the kind of work she does "transformational nourishment."

We can simplify mealtimes by

eating less at each sitting, limiting

the choice of foods we consume,

and not going back for seconds.

Eating consciously also requires that we tune in to our own internal rhythms by slowing down before mealtimes, which might include escaping for a few moments to unwind between work and dinner, turning off the television to enjoy the silence, taking a collective moment of silence at the table, or simply saying a few words of gratitude before we dig in. It also means getting in sync with nature by eating fresh seasonal foods that connect us with the earth; instead of eating pineapples in the winter that have been frozen and shipped, take a trip to your local farmer's market to discover what's growing. And when you find yourself mindlessly opening the refrigerator or going straight for the sugar, Schatz recommends asking yourself, *Who are you feeding?* to get to the root of these ingrained impulses.

Mindful eating has one last requirement: dropping our neurotic thinking about food. "We have to be realistic," says Schatz. "It doesn't mean that we can't ever have chocolate or coffee; it just means that the day-to-day nourishment practice is well engaged, and the regular practice of feeding ourselves is one of intention, respect, and love. And from that place, we arrive as a much more whole individual."

More important, we can learn to listen to our bodies. If we are tired, what are we going to do about it? Many times we think, *That's just how it is.* But it doesn't have to be that way. We can feel good about our bodies, feel healthy and vital, and also get things done in the world.

Going on a retreat, taking time to nourish our bodies, cleansing our bodies of toxins through fasting, and doing an emotional cleansing are all things we can do to step off the busy treadmill of our lives and regain our center. But these things often trigger negative feelings of guilt and selfishness. A woman in overdrive might think: *How can I go away and leave my husband to take care of the kids? How can I spend X number of dollars on a weekend getaway when we need it for the family's next vacation?* So much of our lives requires a delicate balancing act. Juggling work and home life. Juggling friends and responsibilities. Juggling our personal needs with the needs of our families. It's helpful to take a step back to look at the benefits: a cool head, a calm mind, and an open heart.

Retreats

Most women in overdrive fantasize about getting away from it all. Stepping completely off the treadmill to reconnect with our natural state of balance requires some planning, but it's not impossible to do; I knew one woman with five children of all ages who took off for a week! When it comes to self-reflection, each of us responds to circumstances differently. Are we most at peace while meditating at a Zen center, rock climbing in the high desert, or practicing gentle yoga? Or maybe we'd rather commune with nature in a Costa Rican jungle or work out muscular tension on the massage table. Luckily, there seem to be getaways that suit all these preferences, and more. Hundreds of retreat centers exist, with more opening each week. Here are a few that I've found to be the best. Each supports you in restoring a run-down body, rejuvenating a tired spirit, and ultimately bringing you into better alignment with your inner truth, clarity, and wisdom.

Canyon Ranch
Tucson, Arizona

This crown jewel of spas— which offers dozens of enticing and unusual massages, facials, and body treatments—will also help you establish a personalized program for improved health for years to come. The ranch offers a menu of wellness services like bone density testing and antioxidant evaluation, as well as an impressive roster of on-site doctors, therapists, acupuncturists, and nutritionists.

www.canyonranch.com

Esalen Institute

Big Sur, California

Perched along twenty-seven acres of California's Big Sur, Esalen's abundant grounds include a five-acre working garden, arts center, and its famed cliffside baths, which have been lovingly restored in recent years. The institute, which pioneered the Human Potential Movement in the 1960s, now offers more than four hundred eclectic workshops a year taught by experts in the spirituality, psychology, and health fields.

www.esalen.org

Feathered Pipe Ranch

Helena, Montana

Thousands of dedicated yogis retreat to this Montana mountain paradise to learn from the world's best teachers. The ranch also offers massage, acupuncture, craniosacral therapy, acupressure, and energy work to relieve sore muscles and rejuvenate—a welcome addition after a day of intensive, exhilarating, and sometimes exhausting yoga sessions.

www.featheredpipe.com

Kripalu Center for Yoga & Health

Lenox, Massachusetts

An openhearted and peaceful philosophy infuses every aspect of this beloved Berkshires retreat. Whether you come for one of hundreds of diverse workshops or just a little rest and relaxation, you'll find an unusually talented staff of body workers, daily classes in yoga and meditation, and serene grounds that invite introspection.

www.kripalu.org

Maya Tulum

Tulum, Mexico

It's tempting not to leave your seaside cabana at Maya Tulum, but you'll be glad you did. This Yucatan Peninsula resort offers daily yoga classes, an array of spa and body treatments, and water-based adventures like snorkeling, diving, and boat trips. And if the thought of planning the trip itself induces stress, sign up for the all-inclusive Mind Body Spirit Program—all you have to do is show up.

www.mayatulum.com

Miraval

Catalina, Arizona

Miraval offers pampering with a purpose: bringing your stress levels into check. To this end, this desert resort offers the best of massage and spa treatments and a dizzying number of highly specialized daily classes in yoga, meditation, adventure, creative arts, and nutrition. Check out "The Spirit of Tea," "Mindful Eating," "Create and Rejuvenate with Clay," and "Equine Experience."

www.miravalresort.com

Omega Institute

Rhinebeck, New York

The cream of the crop from the yoga, holistic health, and spiritual worlds come to teach workshops at this homey upstate New York center. Whether you are taking a workshop or want to de-stress with some solo time, you can take daily yoga classes, wander to the lake, explore the tranquil grounds, and visit the dedicated meditation space for some inner—and outer—quiet.

www.eomega.com

Pura Vida Wellness Retreat & Spa

San Jose, Costa Rica

At Pura Vida, which is located on a lush mountaintop in Costa Rica, you'll find tranquility among the center's enchanting gardens, during an indulgent treatment at the wellness center, or simply while lying on the hammock and gazing at the abundant wildlife and natural beauty before you.

www.puravidaspa.com

Rancho La Puerta

Tecate, Mexico

Travelers from around the world migrate to this unrivaled health spa—set against the backdrop of a sacred mountain—for its thriving organic garden; à la carte spa treatments; classes in yoga, meditation, and tai chi; and über-mellow atmosphere. If you prefer action to stillness, choose from one of Rancho's forty daily fitness classes.

www.rancholapuerta.com

The Raj Ayurveda Health Spa

Fairfield, Iowa

Known as the only place besides India to offer an extensive array of traditional techniques of ayurveda—an ancient medical method of preventative care and purification—The Raj promotes inner and outer cleansing through daily detox treatments, yoga and meditation classes, and meticulously prepared and superhealthy meals.

www.theraj.com

Red Mountain Spa

St. George, Utah

If intense physical activity gets you closer to enlightenment, head to Red Mountain. Specializing in hiking, biking, and rock-climbing trips among Moab's stunning rock formations, lava caves, and desert terrain, Red Mountain also offers full-service spa, massage, and body treatments to indulge in after all that exertion.

www.redmountainspa.com

Purple Valley Yoga Centre

Goa, India

Purple Valley, set in a tranquil spot on the western coast of India, caters to nomadic spiritual seekers. After taking a class at the center's charming yoga studio, visitors can meander to a nearby massage hut, tropical gardens, and Buddhist meditation center for some quiet contemplation.

www.yogagoa.net

Samasati Nature Retreat

Puerto Viejo, Costa Rica

Claim your bungalow at Samasati, an eco-resort and retreat center on 250 acres of tropical rainforest overlooking the Caribbean sea. Here you can retreat with a specific yoga teacher, receive Reiki or shiatsu, and contemplate the vastness of the natural world on a hike, bird-watch, or swim with the dolphins.

www.samasati.com

Shambhala Mountain Center

Red Feather Lakes. Colorado

Perched eight thousand feet above sea level, this Rocky Mountain refuge offers an array of workshops on Tibetan Buddhist meditation and philosophy, yoga retreats, and personal getaways. Global travelers flock to see the 108-foot-tall Great Stupa of Dharmakaya, a sacred architectural wonder filled with original art and sculpture and considered the only one of its kind in North America.

www.shambhalamountain.org

Tensing Pen Hotel

Negril. Jamaica

Receiving an oceanside massage, eating in an open-air kitchen, and sleeping in a thatched-roof cottage are all highly likely scenarios at Jamaica's Tensing Pen, a Tibetan-influenced locale on the western tip of Jamaica whose delightfully remote setting is optimal for downtime and introspection.

www.tensingpen.com

words
to live
by

I'll be turning thirty-four soon. I've had my first child. For the first time, my husband and I are going to see a financial advisor. As we've begun thinking about saving for a college fund, the age spots on my arms seem suddenly more pronounced. My knees hurt for no apparent reason. I have stray gray hairs. Suddenly, I'm saying things like, "I knew you fifteen years ago, in college." In other words, I'm aging.

One interesting thing I've learned while writing this book is that no one really feels her age. Women who are fifty feel thirty-five. Women on the verge of receiving Social Security feel fifty.

The concept of aging is moving from something dreaded to something accepted. A 2005 Harris Interactive survey, done in conjunction with the International Longevity Center (ILC), on attitudes about aging in the United States found that a majority of Americans hold positive views on aging and older persons. The study found that most people do not agree with recent claims that older persons place an undue burden on society. The survey gauges the views of American adults regarding the capacity of older persons to learn, work, and remain productive. With the projected doubling of the older population by 2025, the first of the Baby Boomers turning sixty this year, Social Security, as well as Medicare and retirement age, reform at the forefront of policy and labor discussions, and reports of age discrimination in the workforce and in medical treatment, it is particularly critical to assess the public's views on older people and aging, and its correlation to institutional ageism.

Key findings of this Harris/ILC survey include the following:

→ A total of 92 percent of all adults do not agree that older persons are a burden on society. Eighty-one percent disagree with the claim that older people receive more than their fair share of benefits with Medicare and Social Security.

→ The majority of Americans view older persons as active members of the labor force. About eight in ten of all adults (79 percent) believe that older workers are as productive as younger workers, and that older workers work as hard as young and middle-aged workers (83 percent).[1]

But don't take mere statistics as evidence that aging is becoming a more positive experience. As a woman in overdrive, I have wondered whether I will ever get off the track of being a superwoman. The good news, though, is that the women I spoke with have embraced their aging process in different ways over the decades of their lives—and learned valuable lessons about themselves and the world along the way. Women told me that they feel stronger, more confident, and in better shape as they age. They shared with me that they still feel young, healthy, sexy, and vibrant well into their older years. And their stories about dealing with stress, overdrive, and aging gracefully have been inspiring and fascinating. Here are a few.

Women told me that they feel stronger,

more confident, and in better shape

as they age. They shared with me that

they still feel young, healthy, sexy, and

vibrant well into their older years.

The Thirties

Colleen Morton Busch, age thirty-six, novelist
I don't feel like I'm old now—I think the thirties are considered young—but then somehow when you turn forty you are all of a sudden old, or perceived as old, by society. I've always thought that's strange. So I'm not exactly looking forward to turning forty. By contrast, I was delighted to turn thirty and oh so happy to be done with my twenties—to be a grown-up woman! I hang around a lot of people older than me, including my husband, so I get to feel perpetually young and get teased for being the youngest. But when I'm around my friends' kids, the ones who have teenagers and kids in college, I have this funny feeling. I realize that they consider me old! I don't feel old at all, but I know that to them thirty-six is old.

Inside I feel at my strongest physically. I'm in better shape than I was even in my twenties. I don't feel slowed down in any way. I feel calmer, less intense emotionally, and I guess that's probably an effect of aging. I feel somewhat settled, or dropped into, the rhythm of my life. I am basically comfortable with myself and can ride out self-esteem storms more skillfully than I could when I was younger. Sometimes I do long for that intensity, however. I once heard someone say they didn't write poems anymore like they did when they were young because they weren't as brave as they were then. I know what they mean. Though I didn't consider writing poetry a particularly brave act when I was getting my MFA in poetry in my twenties and writing lots of poems, now I think it is and was courageous. Back then I didn't care what I was going to do beyond my degree. I just wanted to write good poems.

Advice for someone in her twenties: I think it's true that youth is wasted on the young. You just don't have the sense of your own immortality and the transience of things to appreciate the gifts of youth. But I'd say: Don't be in such a hurry to grow up. It will happen. Don't worry about what others think. Do what you dream about doing, and if you don't have dreams, cultivate them. Keep friends of all ages—it's good for perspective. Take care of your skin (sunscreen, and I particularly recommend facials at least seasonally) and your body. Don't stay in relationships that hurt you or drive you crazy -there really are more fish in the sea.

Cyndy Brannvall, age thirty-nine, massage therapist
It's hard to separate "aging" from the culmination of my experience overall. The last few years, I think I have just started to feel like I am getting older; I would describe that as having had significant life experiences: getting married and divorced, losing my parents, dealing with my aging grandmother, beginning the empty-nest transition, losing the battle of the bulge, having a noticeable amount of gray hair and odd allergy and skin conditions that I never had before. But other than that, I feel the same inside, even richer. Maybe I'm a more refined version of who I have always been.

Having had my daughter when I was twenty-three, my overdrive years were in my twenties and early thirties when I was working full-time; doing everything for my small child; trying to maintain a healthy, loving connection with my partner; and thinking that I could also go to school, get a degree, exercise,

Don't be in such a hurry to grow up. It will happen. Don't worry about what others think. Do what you dream about doing, and if you don't have dreams, cultivate them.

and have time to pursue the hobbies that feed my soul. Now that I am actually getting older, my life seems to be opening up. I have a career that has enabled me to be primarily focused on raising my daughter. She is now sixteen and becoming independent in leaps and bounds, so I'm not driving her everywhere, cleaning up after her, etc. She's learning to do all of that sort of stuff for herself, so I have some spaciousness in my life. I'm in transition to moving some of my focus and energy back to myself.

I've had to make choices. I found that I couldn't be a super-woman. I guess the negative was that I wasn't able to invest in getting an education for myself and that I've worked in jobs that I didn't really like at times. I feel like I've been "just making it" financially for a long time, and I'm really sick of that. On the positive side, my life was so chaotic that I started doing meditation every day. That turned out to be a really positive thing; it enabled me to really be present with my daughter and my life. I was able to switch gears from working all the time and being productive to playing Barbies or taking an hour and a half to walk around the block with my three-year-old, looking at worms and puddles and drops of water on plants. And to be okay with the house being a mess and spending an entire day sitting in the yard making daisy chains and playing fairy with my daughter and her friend. So I was poor, but I don't feel like I missed the important stuff.

I did have a bit of conflict with the women's lib thing in a certain way, and with my girlfriends of that era. I sort of felt like, "Thanks a lot!" Now I get to do all of the house stuff, child stuff, *and* I'm expected to work full-time and have a high-powered career. Thanks, but no thanks. My friends who were there paving the way for my generation feel that I take for granted the opportunities that I have available, and that I don't appreciate what they did for me. I do appreciate it. I just think we (as women) are still refining it to get it right.

The Forties

Keren Taylor, age forty-one, executive director of WriteGirl
Aging gracefully means accepting aging, not fighting it, and allowing it to show on your body, mind, and pace. To fight it is to be very ungraceful about something that is a natural progression—it doesn't have to be downward. I'm starting to do more hiking, and I might be in better cardiovascular shape that I was at thirty. I still feel invigorated. I've always admired that gray-haired woman who looks so beautiful but has a different pace or sense of life around her.

Now that I am in early menopause, I'm much better able to approach it with a sense of humor. That's part of aging gracefully—to see the light and the beauty of aging and the really great things that come with age, like knowledge and the wisdom of not making the same mistake twice. You couldn't pay me to go back to my twenties and all of the inexperience that comes with it.

I would advise a younger woman to take advantage of the energy that you have. You can stay up late and get up early! Don't destroy that energy with too much drinking. That energy is really your creative energy that allows you to create things of beauty, so use it and think about where you can put it and what

Aging gracefully means accepting

aging, not fighting it, and allowing it to

show on your body, mind, and pace.

you want to channel. That energy that seems boundless and endless can create something of magic and joy for those around you. Don't waste it. At forty you'll go, "Gee, why didn't I think of painting or starting a nonprofit when I had the energy and the time?" The biggest change has been my level of energy. It's sort of disheartening. You feel like your life energy seeps away from you, and when I was younger I didn't feel that way. I am working so hard and am so focused, my days are so full, I'm challenging myself and meeting people, and it's extremely challenging. I'm completely tapped out. Although I don't have the energy that I used to have, there are other things that I have that I never used to have—like wisdom.

Laura Glynn, age forty-six, legal secretary

As a woman, in a way you *have* to be a superwoman to keep everything going. On the positive side, this has given me the gift to have all of these relationships in every area and to pour out positive things I've learned. I can help out the older generation, like my mom, and that definitely has been positive. On the negative side, you have to make sure that you can grab that time for yourself to get pumped up to keep giving, or else you crash and burn.

It's a very interesting time of my life. Since I've turned around forty-three, I have a new burst of energy. I don't know what happens during menopause. People say they get all aggressive, but I've found that it's enhanced me. I'm running, learning to surf, and I feel so energized. This helps me to get time by myself and strengthen my body for this next section of life that I'm entering. It's interesting because here I am, getting older, and I'm more fit and toned than I was when having children. I know other women who are doing workouts like never before. It's a good way to give positive energy. When I run it gives me time to get centered and get focused.

I would tell younger women to start working out right now, and after you have children work out. Physiologically, your body does all of these crazy things during each decade of your life, and I never knew that.

Remember the old adage, "Take each day slowly and drink it in, and appreciate those around you." It all goes so fast. I listened to this advice and it *still* went too fast.

To cope with overdrive, I would say take some time in the mornings.

People say they don't have time, but I used to invite my children to sit with me while I read the Bible or prayed. It's so important to make time, even twenty minutes. Use your community, friends, or spouse to say, "I've got to take a forty-five-minute bath."

I guess I have a delightfully positive view about aging. A few years ago, when I saw wrinkles and a gray hair, I told my husband I feel like the Velveteen Rabbit. I've had a life well lived and well loved.

The Fifties

MaryAnn Gray, age fifty, social psychologist
Looking back, I realize that I spent way too much time in the sun! I knew I was hurting my skin, but I only cared about how I looked that night. I would change that. I would try to create a fitness regimen earlier. Psychologically, or personally—because of my own experience of trauma at a very young age—I was afraid to do a lot. I have lived a life with way too much fear. I can't blame my family, but what happened exacerbated and hardened that fear.

It's easy to say that I wish it took me until now to feel confident enough to take some small risks in life. I'm not a risk-taker and I never will be. I am now trying to write a book, and until now I've been too afraid of failing, feeling pain, and upsetting people.

I don't know if it will succeed, but it's what I want to do. I can't control my success or failure, but I can control the effort that I make. Some people learn that at an earlier age. I'll never be a risk-taker, although I wish that I had the support and temperament.

Zoe Elton, age fifty-four, film festival programmer
You must do what you love. You must do what your heart tells you to do. It's really that simple. When you connect with the things that you love, your spirit just flies. That is what you are supposed to be doing. It's very easy to feel guilty about things that aren't important.

There is so much focus on achievement. I have a goddaughter in London; she is very smart and goes to a school with smart kids. She was having problems with her reading comprehension homework, and we were talking about it and she said, "It's my mind tripping me up." It was something that she didn't love, but she said, "I know I have to get good grades, get into university, get a good job, and make a lot of money." But that's not true. I didn't know what to say to her. I had kids whom I taught in London and then who, for one reason or another, didn't necessarily go the route of good job and good exams. The truth is, they are all artists, so if you are a creative person, that kind of stuff doesn't matter.

Sherry Astmann, age fifty-nine, product manager
Everyone handles stress differently. A person who is a homemaker may feel totally overwhelmed. It has a lot to do with your basic nature. I'm very high energy and always have been a working mom. I was also a single mom for a lot of the time my kids were growing up. So I've always thought, *Okay, this is the way it is.*

Being a single mom made it harder than anything, emotionally, to have the kids and to do it all by myself. Becky, my younger daughter, had special needs, so I wasn't just coming home, making dinner, and making sure the kids had a bath. I had to run her around all over the place. Quite frankly, I don't think someone with less energy could've done that. It was really intense. The kids were latchkey kids. I'm not going to kid anybody and say that it was easy. There is nothing harder than having an infant, the physicality of it all. As the kids got older, it became more emotional, to have to worry about drugs and alcohol and drinking and driving.

My advice is to live each moment and not sweat the small stuff. There is so much that is bigger and more important in life than a new pair of shoes or a car. Getting older is something to look forward to. I feel like I'm in a really good place in my head right now. Try to learn something new every day, even if it's really simple, like the meaning of a word. It gets boring when you stop learning.

Be a good role model: Live your life in a way that you would want your children to live their lives. One of the things that I taught my girls is to always shake hands firmly. It shows confidence. I think it tells a lot about you. You should also smile and laugh when you are stressed. You have to try to find the humor somewhere, and you may have to work really hard and know that everything happens for a reason.

Getting older is something to look forward to.

Try to learn something new every day, even

if it's really simple, like the meaning of a

word. It gets boring when you stop learning.

The Sixties

Terry Ferretti, age sixty-one, wife, mother, grandmother
You really can never stop learning. Keep doing things that keep your mind active, like card playing and dancing. I went back to dancing and had the best year of my life. It helped me get through a grieving process after my sister died.

I'm not going to age gracefully. I'm going kicking, fighting, and screaming! I always used to tell people my age, but I don't do that anymore. People treat you differently. You get isolated from social groups. I know I am the same person I was, but if they hear you are over sixty, they think you are over the hill. I don't want to be treated like I'm old.

I was a feminist in the 1960s; I have two daughters and I always wanted them to have opportunities that men have. It's mind-boggling to someone like me who witnessed things like the first female in medical school.

Be patient when going through difficult times; sometimes it just takes life to get through things. There are some things that only age, growth, and wisdom can see you through. Try to have something spiritual in your life—life is tough, and you need it to get through that. Nurture family, friends, and faith.

Carol Shapiro, age sixty-six, yoga and meditation teacher
I see my life divided into almost different lifetimes. My first role was as a daughter and sister. There was a lot of pressure put on me and the message that I wasn't smart enough, so that phase of my life kind of fueled the rest of my life and becoming a superwoman. I went to a college that was probably a little

more difficult than I could handle, so that was another honing of that image. I had been raised in retail business, and my father brought me up from the time I was very young to learn the business.

By the time I graduated from high school, I was a buyer and knew all there was to know about retailing. I got a liberal arts degree and majored in English literature. When I got out of school, I was engaged to a medical student. I was an assistant buyer for three years before my husband decided we should have a child.

I was a stay-at-home mom, which I don't regret. Part of being a superwoman is being a stay-at-home mom. Unless you've been home all the time with children, I don't think you can understand what the responsibilities are and what the mental challenges can be. That was difficult for me at times, when both of my kids were in nursery school and first grade. I started taking classes at the botanical gardens. I seemed to have an aptitude for plants and horticulture, and this was the next phase of my life. It put more stress on me because I put too much pressure on myself, but it also made me aware that I have capabilities that I didn't think I had, realize that I can manage several things at one time, and know that if a job needs to be done I can usually get it done.

It's a really different world now—a world of cell phones and computers. The technology is so different, and there is so much more to juggle and so much more stimulus. I would say choose to be selective about the amount of stimuli in your life to keep your life at a reasonable pace, which would mean constantly asking yourself, *How can I simplify?*

It's never too soon to be conscious of diet and exercise. It's really important that these are factors in your life that have a profound effect on aging. Too often younger women are so busy that these are not priorities, there isn't time to select healthy food, and so you grab whatever is available. There isn't time to work in time for aerobic exercise, yoga, and healthy eating, and this is so important.

Faith Isaacs, age sixty-four, yoga teacher and grandmother
I asked my mom about aging and what she would've liked to know. She said a few things about traveling more and a regular meditation practice. Then she said: "I wish I was more conscious and more spiritually self-aware, knowing there is more to life than what you just see, feel, and hear."

I've thought a lot about that statement over the past few weeks, since I know my life is about to change radically. I wonder how I will handle the sleepless nights and the selfless devotion it takes to raise a child. I wonder if I will be able to continue to lead a balanced life and take time out for myself while caring for my newborn. I wonder if I will feel the pressure to become a woman in overdrive without stopping to enjoy the simple pleasures or the present moment.

Make the Choice

After talking to so many women during the course of this book, I realize that living consciously and with spiritual awareness is a choice. By living this way, I can choose to age gracefully, live in a balanced way, and stay conscious of my effect on those around

It's never too soon to be conscious of diet

and exercise. Too often younger women

are so busy that these are not priorities,

there isn't time to select healthy food,

and so you grab whatever is available.

me. I can learn to use each experience as an opportunity for growth, knowing that becoming an aware human being doesn't happen sitting alone on a mountaintop, but during daily interactions with our spouses, friends, children, and communities. And I know that I can count on the advice and inspiration from generations of women who have walked the path before me. By listening to their words of wisdom, I have learned that I can choose to accept the days when I'm crying tears of frustration as easily as the days filled with perfect bliss. I can go into overdrive when necessary and I can pull back when it gets to be too much. I can align myself with the flow of the world and allow life to happen the way it's going to happen, without fear or resistance. And this newfound knowledge is a relief and a blessing.

Resource Guide

Books

30 Essential Yoga Poses: For Beginning Students and Their Teachers,
by Judith Lasater (Rodmell, 2003)

After the Ecstasy, the Laundry: How the Heart Grows Wise on the Spiritual Path, by Jack Kornfield (Bantam, 2001)

Age Erasers for Women: Actions You Can Take Right Now to Look Younger and Feel Great, edited by Patricia Fisher (Rodale 1994)

The Ancient Cookfire, by Carrie L'Esperance (Bear & Company, 1998)

The Artist's Way: A Spiritual Path to Higher Creativity, by Julia Cameron (Tarcher, 2002)

Being Peace, by Thich Nhat Hanh (Parallax, 1987)

Bird by Bird: Some Instructions on Writing and Life, by Anne Lamott (Anchor, 1995)

Consciously Female: How to Listen to Your Body and Your Soul for a Lifetime of Healthier Living, by Tracy W. Gaudet, MD, with Paula Spencer and Andrew M. Weil (Bantam, 2004)

Emotional Intelligence: Why It Can Matter More Than IQ, by Daniel Goleman (Bantam, 1995)

Faith: Trusting Your Own Deepest Experience, by Sharon Salzberg (Riverhead, 2002)

Living Your Yoga: Finding the Spiritual in Everyday Life, by Judith Lasater (Rodmell Press, 1999)

Lovingkindness: The Revolutionary Art of Happiness, by Sharon Salzberg (Shambhala, 1997)

Mother Nurture: A Mother's Guide to Health in Body, Mind, and Intimate Relationships, by Rick Hanson, PhD, Jan Hanson, L.Ac., and Ricki Pollycove, MD (Penguin, 2002)

Not Your Mother's Midlife: A Ten-Step Guide to Fearless Aging,
by Nancy Alspaugh and Marilyn Kentz (Andrews McMeel, 2003)

The Overspent American: Why We Want What We Don't Need,
by Juliet B. Schor (Harper, 1999)

The Overworked American: The Unexpected Decline of Leisure,
by Juliet B. Schor (Basic, 1993)

The Path of Practice: A Woman's Book of Healing with Food, Breath, and Sound, by Bri. Maya Tiwari (Ballantine, 2000)

Perfect Balance: Dr. Robert Greene's Breakthrough Program for Finding the Lifelong Hormonal Health You Deserve, by Robert A. Greene, MD, and Leah Feldon (Clarkson Potter, 2005)

Positive Energy: 10 Extraordinary Prescriptions for Transforming Fatigue, Stress & Fear into Vibrance, Strength and Love, by Judith Orloff, MD (Three Rivers/Random House 2004)

Relax and Renew: Restful Yoga for Stressful Times, by Judith Lasater, PhD (Rodmell Press, 1995)

The Relaxation Response, by Herbert Benson (HarperTorch, 1976)

Slow Your Clock Down: The Complete Guide to a Healthy, Younger You, by Judith Reichman, MD (William Morrow, 2004)

Voluntary Simplicity: Toward a Way of Life That Is Outwardly Simple, Inwardly Rich, by Duane Elgin (William Morrow, 1981)

The Wisdom of No Escape: And the Path of Loving Kindness,
by Pema Chödrön (Shambhala, 2001)

Writing Down the Bones: Freeing the Writer Within,
by Natalie Goldberg (Shambhala, 1986)

Yoga and the Quest for the True Self, by Stephen Cope (Bantam, 1999)

Yoga: The Spirit and Practice of Moving into Stillness,
by Erich Schiffmann (Pocket, 1996)

Your Money or Your Life: Transforming Your Relationship with Money and Achieving Financial Independence, by Joe Dominguez and Vicki Robin (Viking, 1992)

Websites

www.DrWeil.com
Alternative doctor Dr. Andrew Weil's comprehensive website.

www.healthjourneys.com
Complete guide to guided-imagery CDs and information.

www.healthywomen.org
Website of the nonprofit National Women's Health Resource Center.

www.nccam.nih.gov
National Center for Complementary and Alternative Medicine's official website.

www.nlm.nih.gov
The United States National Library of Medicine.

www.WebMD.com
Search by condition or symptom.

www.wholehealthmd.com
Complementary and alternative medicine education and information.

Magazines and Journals

Alternative Medicine
www.alternativemedicine.com

Alternative Therapies in Health and Medicine
www.alternative-therapies.com

Natural Health
www.naturalhealthmag.com

Journal of the American Medical Association
http://jama.ama-assn.org/collections

Shambhala Sun
www.shambhalasun.com

Tricycle
www.tricycle.com

Yoga Journal
www.yogajournal.com

Yoga International
www.himalayaninstitute.org/yogaplus

Organizations

Chopra Center
www.chopra.com

Kripalu Center for Yoga & Health
www.kripalu.org

Omega Institute
www.Eomega.com

The Slow Movement
www.slowmovement.com

Notes

Introduction

1. RIC media relations. Found online at: www.ric.org/about/news/pr_display. php?id=140.

Chapter 1: Combating Low Energy: Brain Drain and Body Blues

1. Patricia Fisher, ed. *Age Erasers for Women: Actions You Can Take Right Now to Look Younger and Feel Great* (New York: St. Martin's, 1994), 163.

2. Rick Hanson, Jan Hanson, and Ricki Pollycove. *Mother Nurture* (New York: Penguin, 2002), 1.

3. Ibid, 336.

4. Calley O'Neill, in conversation with the author.

5. MaryAnn Gray, in conversation with the author.

6. Robert A. Greene, MD, and Leah Feldon. *Perfect Balance: Dr. Robert Greene's Breakthrough Program for Finding the Lifelong Hormonal Health You Deserve* (New York: Clarkson Potter, 2005), 236.

7. Ibid, 235.

8. MacArthur Foundation Study on Aging, cited in Dr. Andrew Weil's article in *Body & Soul*. Specific details can be obtained from the following two studies:
1. Seeman TE, Berkman LF, Charpentier P, Blazer D, Albert M, Tinetti M. "Behavioral and Psychosocial Predictors of Physical Performance: MacArthur Studies of Successful Aging." *Journal of Gerontology* 50A: M177–M183, 1995.
2. Albert MS, Jones K, Savage CR, Berkman L, Seeman T, Blazer D, Rowe JW. "Predictors of Cognitive Change in Older Persons: MacArthur Studies of Successful Aging." *Psychology and Aging* 10: 578–589, 1995.

9. Terry Ferretti, in conversation with the author.

10. CDC study. Found online at: www.cdc.gov/cfs or www.webmd.com/hw /brain_nervous_system/nord416.asp.

11. Chronic Fatigue Syndrome Information Resources. Found online at: www.niaid .nih.gov/factsheets/cfs.htm#5.

12. "Genetics and Stress Are Found Linked to Fatigue Disorder" in *The New York Times*, April 21, 2006. Found online at: www.nytimes.com/2006/04/21/health /21fatigue.html?ex=1303272000&en=ffe1c3f3aa02a311&ei=5088&partner =rssnyt&emc=rss.

Chapter 2: Cultivating Slowness and Relaxation

1. In Praise of Slow. Found online at: www.inpraiseofslow.com/slow/faq.php.

2. Humphrey Taylor. "Reading, TV, Spending Time with Family, Gardening and Fishing Top List of Favorite Leisure-Time Activities." Harris Interactive, August 8, 2001. Found online at: www.harrisinteractive.com/harris_poll/index.asp?PID=249.

3. Keren Taylor, in conversation with the author.

4. U.S. Department of Labor statistics. Found online at: www.dol.gov/wb/stats/ main.htm.

5. Patricia Fisher, ed. *Age Erasers for Women: Actions You Can Take Right Now to Look Younger and Feel Great* (New York: St. Martin's, 1994), 530.

6. Ibid, 531.

7. Duane Elgin. *Voluntary Simplicity* (New York: Perennial, 1998), 25.

8. Ibid.

Chapter 3: Squelching Stress and Elevating the Spirit

1. The name has been changed in this story.

2. Xenia Montenegro. "The Divorce Experience: A Study of Divorce at Midlife and Beyond." *AARP The Magazine,* May 2004. Found online at: www.aarp.org/research/reference/publicopinions/aresearch-import-867.html.

3. The National Center for Health Statistics, part of the federal Centers for Disease Control and Prevention. Found online at: www.cdc.gov/nchs/pressroom/05facts /prelimbirths04.htm.

4. Andrew Weil. "Can Spirituality Heal?" Dr. Andrew Weil's Self Healing, January 2000. Found online at: www.ajph.org/cgi/content/abstract/

5. Mark Twain quote. Found online at: http://en.wikiquote.org/wiki/Mark_Twain.

6. Daniel Goleman. *Emotional Intelligence: Why It Can Matter More Than IQ* (New York: Bantam, 1995).

7. Bri. Maya Tiwari. *The Path of Practice: A Woman's Book of Ayurvedic Healing* (New York: Wellspring/Ballantine, 2001), 5.

Chapter 4: Capturing Longevity

1. David Ewing Duncan. "Finding the Fountain of Youth" in the *San Francisco Chronicle Sunday Magazine,* May 29, 2005. Found online at: www.sfgate.com.

2. MacArthur Foundation Study. Found online at: www.helpguide.org/aging_well.htm.

3. Judith Reichman, MD. *Slow Your Clock Down: The Complete Guide to a Healthy, Younger You* (New York: William Morrow, 2004), 310.

4. Ibid.

5. Ibid.

6. Source: American Society of Plastic Surgeons. Found online at: www.plasticsurgery.org/news_room/press_releases/2005-procedural-stats.cfm.

7. Monika White, Center for Healthy Aging, in conversation with the author.

Chapter 5: Understanding Complementary and Alternative Medicine

1. AARP Research Center. Found online at: www.aarp.org/research/health/healthquality/aresearch-import-722-IB46.html.

2. "The Use of Complementary and Alternative Medicine in the United States." National Center for Complementary and Alternative Medicine. Found online at: http://nccam.nih.gov/news/camsurvey_fs1.htm#use.

3. Tracey W. Gaudet, MD. *Consciously Female: How to Listen to Your Body and Your Soul for a Lifetime of Healthier Living* (New York: Bantam, 2004), 28–29.

4. "What Is Complementary and Alternative Medicine." National Center for Complementary and Alternative Medicine. Found online at: http://nccam.nih.gov/health/whatiscam/.

5. Ibid.

6. Ibid.

7. Women's Health America. Found online at: www.womenshealth.com/pms.html.

8. Robert A. Greene, MD, and Leah Feldon. *Perfect Balance: Dr. Robert Greene's Breakthrough Program for Finding the Lifelong Hormonal Health You Deserve* (New York: Clarkson Potter, 2005), 206–07.

9. Patricia Fisher, ed. *Age Erasers for Women: Actions You Can Take Right Now to Look Younger and Feel Great* (New York: St. Martin's, 1994), 292.

10. "Depression: Depression in Women." Web MD. Found online at: www.webmd.com/content/article/46/1663_51233.htm.

Chapter 6: Discovering Mind/Body Exercises

1. "Mind/Body Health: Did You Know?" American Psychological Association. Found online at: www.apahelpcenter.org/articles/article.php?id=103.

2. Pema Chödrön. *The Wisdom of No Escape: And the Path of Loving Kindness* (Berkeley, CA: Shambhala, 2001), 3.

Chapter 7: Restoring the Body During Sickness and Disease

1. U.S. Department of Labor statistics. Found online at: www.bls.gov/opub/ted/2000/feb/wk3/art03.htm.

2. "Breast Cancer: Overview of Breast Cancer." Web MD. Found online at: www.webmd.com/content/article/9/1662_52440.htm.

3. Dana Davies, consultant, Blue Cross, in conversation with the author.

Chapter 8: Finding Hormonal Balance

1. "Women's Health Initiative on HRT Stopped," September 24, 2002. HRT study from Yale-New Haven Hospital. Found online at: www.ynhh.org/healthlink/womens/womens_9_02.html.

2. Herbert Benson, MD, and Miriam Z. Klipper. *The Relaxation Response* (New York: Avon Books, 1975), 72.

3. "Turning Lemons into Lemonade: Hardiness Helps People Turn Stressful Circumstances into Opportunities." APA study. Found online at: www.psychologymatters.org/hardiness.html.

4. "Americans Engage in Unhealthy Behaviors to Manage Stress." APA survey, February 23, 2006. Found online at: http://apahelpcenter.mediaroom.com/index.php?s=press_releases&item=23.

5. "Chronic Exposure to Stress Hormone Causes Anxious Behavior in Mice, Confirming the Mechanism by Which Long-term Stress Can Lead to Mood Disorders." APA press release, April 16, 2006. Found online at: www.apa.org/releases/stressmood0406.html.

Chapter 9: Hop Off the Treadmill

1. Carrie L'Esperance. *The Ancient Cookfire: How to Rejuvenate Body and Spirit Through Seasonal Foods and Fasting* (Santa Fe, NM: Bear & Company, 1998), xxi.

Appendix: Words to Live By

1. International Longevity Center. Found online at: www.ilcusa.org.

Acknowledgments

I've been blessed to have been guided, supported, and loved by a throng of superhumans too numerous to mention and who have contributed both directly and indirectly to this book.

Much gratitude to the following: Brooke Warner for her vision and sharp eye. Allen Salkin for his loyalty and advice, both solicited and unsolicited. Kathryn Arnold for her mentorship and generosity. Judith Hanson Lasater for her eloquence and helping thousands of modern women relax and take it easy. Deborah Byrd and James Woolley for nurturing my interest in writing and women's issues. Linda Loewenthal for sticking with me.

Ross Gay and Andre Lambertson bring light and beauty to the world. Together Scott Schmidt, Chris White, Haui Tarshes, and Susan Nicholas set the stage for creativity and community. Andrea Ferretti, Amy Gerard, and Jessica Scadron are wonderful lifelong friends. Yeshi, Nancy, and Shanthi transform the world with grace.

The Glynn family blesses me with its love and encouragement; I feel so lucky to have the enthusiasm and support of Ephraim, Janice, Kara, and Susannah. And I cherish the love of Bennie, Jim, Lynn, and Jamie.

A big thank you to: the San Francisco Integral Yoga Institute for teaching me the fundamentals; my writer's group for keeping me on my toes; the magazine editors who keep me employed; and my fellow health writers who help raise awareness and nudge about a shift in consciousness through their books and articles.

I can't envision a more loving nuclear family: My sister, Elana, overflows with warmth and compassion and teaches me to believe in magic. Early on, my parents, Michael and Faith, instilled in me the importance of pursuing things intellectual, staying healthy, connecting spiritually, and treating others with kindness. I am eternally grateful for the unconditional love and opportunities they've given me.

My amazing husband, Eric, makes life for a woman in overdrive easy: He runs my business, does most of the housework, takes an equal part in parenting, and loves family life with a passion. He encourages me to dream big, and his partnership provides the solid ground that has helped me bloom. And finally, thank you to the beautiful Lucian Elijah, a gift so great that only God could create.

Index

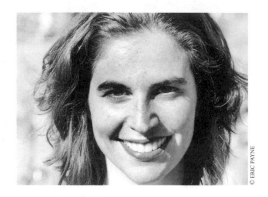

© ERIC PAYNE

About the Author

Nora Isaacs, formerly a senior editor at *Yoga Journal,* is a freelance health journalist and writing coach. Her work has appeared in *Alternative Medicine, Yoga Journal, Body & Soul, Fit Yoga,* Salon.com, *Natural Health,* the *San Francisco Chronicle Magazine*, and many other national and regional publications. Isaacs earned her MA from Columbia School of Journalism. She writes and teaches yoga in San Francisco, where she lives with her husband and baby son.

Credits

Selected Titles from Seal Press

For more than thirty years, Seal Press has published groundbreaking books. By women. For women. Visit our website at www.sealpress.com.

Above Us Only Sky: A Woman Looks Back, Ahead, and into the Mirror by Marion Winik. $14.95. 1-58005-144-8. A witty and engaging book from NPR commentator Marion Winik about facing midlife without getting tangled up in the past or hung up in the future.

A Matter of Choice: 25 People Who Have Transformed Their Lives edited by Joan Chatfield-Taylor. $14.95. 1-58005-118-9. An inspiring collection of essays by people who made profound changes in their work, personal life, location, or lifestyle, proving that it is indeed never too late to take the road less traveled.

Confessions of a Naughty Mommy: How I Found My Lost Libido by Heidi Raykeil. $14.95. 1-58005-157-X. The Naughty Mommy shares her bedroom woes and woo-hoos with other mamas who are rediscovering their sex lives after baby and are ready to think about it, talk about it, and DO it.

Pissed Off: On Women and Anger by Spike Gillespie. $14.95, 1-58005-162-6. An amped-up and personal self-help book that encourages women to go ahead and use that middle finger without being closed off to the notion of forgiveness.

Another Morning: Voices of Truth and Hope From Mothers With Cancer by Linda Blachman. $15.95, 1-58005-178-2. A collection of powerful, inspirational, and deeply moving personal stories of ordinary women responding to every mother's nightmare: a cancer diagnosis while raising children.

What Would Murphy Brown Do? How the Women of Prime Time Changed Our Lives by Allison Klein. $16.95, 1-58005-171-5. From workplace politics to single motherhood and designer heels in the city, revisit TV's favorite—and most influential—women of the 1970s through today who stood up and held their own.